HYPOALLERGENIC DOGS

FACTS & INFORMATION

YOUR COMPLETE GUIDE TO CHOOSING A
HYPOALLERGENIC DOG. INCLUDES
PROFILES ON THE MOST POPULAR
PUREBRED & CROSS BREEDS.

**BY
TIM ANDERSON**

Copyright Information

Acknowledgements

I would like to thank my wife and children for their patience whilst writing this book. Dogs have always been a part of our lives, and our household wouldn't be the same without them. They liven up our home, are always ready to go for a run in the park, and provide a friendly wet nose when you are feeling down.

I was inspired to write this book on hypoallergenic dogs because my two nephews suffer from pet allergies and have a hard time when playing with our dogs. They have always wanted a dog of their own, so hopefully this book can help their parents decide which one would be most suitable for their home and lifestyle.

Dogs featured in photos:

Front Cover (from left): Samoyed, Yorkshire Terrier, Portuguese Water Dog.
Back Cover: Labradoodle
Page 12: Poodle
Page 20: Yorkshire Terrier
Page 36: Labradoodle

All other photos match their corresponding breed profile.

Table of Contents

Table of Contents

Table of Contents

Table of Contents

Table of Contents

Foreword

Dogs...it is just one simple word, but it is a word that is filled with so much. For many, dogs embody everything that is good about life. They are filled with playfulness that brings out our laughter, energy that gets us exercising, and a loyalty that brightens our day when we walk in the door.

They are wonderful companions that bring with them a quiet understanding, a special bond that encourages us to bury our faces into their warm fur when we are at our lowest.

For many people, that warm fur brings sneezing, rashes, and a range of other allergy-related complications. It can be irritating, and while many allergy sufferers love dogs, they either have to heavily medicate themselves to own one or they simply don't own a dog. For people who love dogs, the latter can be torture.

But it doesn't have to be. People with allergies can enjoy life with a dog, and it doesn't have to be one or two dogs. There are dozens of dog breeds that offer hypoallergenic alternatives for allergy sufferers.

In addition, these hypoallergenic dog breeds have a range of personalities, needs, and exercise levels. They can be small and playful or large and quiet. They can be active, lazy, alert, and intelligent. All of the hypoallergenic dog breeds are wonderful creatures that will bring that special bond to everyone in their home -- even those who are suffering from allergies.

This book looks at the most popular hypoallergenic dog breeds that you can purchase and gives you an in-depth view of the breed. By the time you have read through the breed profiles, you will have an understanding of what makes each breed special.

You will also have an understanding of the challenges that each breed has and the pros and cons of the breed. What this means is that you will know whether a breed fits into your home and lifestyle so you can find a perfect match.

All dogs should be a joy to live with, and this goes for hypoallergenic dog breeds. This book is designed to provide you with the understanding you need regarding allergies and overcoming your allergy to dogs.

It will take you through the myths and truths about hypoallergenic dog breeds, how to choose the right breed for you, and also what goes into that hypoallergenic coat. It will also take you through reducing the allergens in your home, regardless of the dog breed that you choose.

Finally, this book will provide you with a list of resources that will help you throughout the life of your pet. The main focus of this book, in fact, was to be a resource for you.

In the end, life is better with a dog. I have created a book that will help you enjoy this wonderful experience. Allergies are a problem we face throughout life, but it doesn't have to be a problem that keeps us from enjoying our pets.

All you need to overcome them is the knowledge to combat the allergens and the perfect canine pooch, and this book will help you with both.

Chapter One: Hypoallergenic?

Although I would love to jump right to the breeds of dogs that are hypoallergenic, it is very important to understand what hypoallergenic is. While many people believe that hypoallergenic means that a dog does not cause allergic reactions in people with allergies, this is not actually the case.

Being hypoallergenic is actually difficult to explain since there are many factors that attribute to the title of hypoallergenic. Because of this, many people end up with dogs that aren't really hypoallergenic, and their allergies suffer.

But it doesn't have to be that way, and in this chapter, I will explain the meaning of hypoallergenic, the myths surrounding the hypoallergenic dog, and the traits that make a dog hypoallergenic.

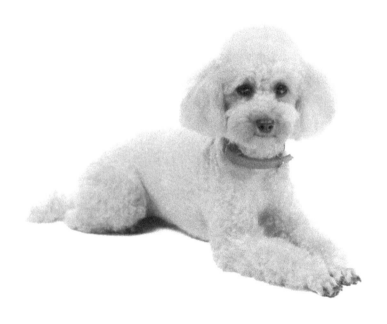

1. The Meaning of Hypoallergenic

The definition of hypoallergenic, when found in the dictionary, is below normal or a slight chance of causing an allergic reaction. It was commonly used in regards to materials that are worn against the skin.

With that in mind, when we apply it to pets, dogs in particular, the word hypoallergenic refers to any animal that has a lower chance of triggering an allergic reaction. This means that there is still a chance of an individual having an allergic reaction, but it is less likely to occur.

One point to mention is that allergens are believed to be connected to one gene. This gene produces a protein that is found on the dog, or animal, and is the cause of the allergic reaction.

Dogs that are considered hypoallergenic lack this particular gene or they produce only small amounts of the protein, which reduces the amount of allergen that can cause a reaction in an allergy sufferer.

There are many breeds that are considered hypoallergenic; however, it is important to look at each individual allergy sufferer. While there may be a dog breed that works with one person's allergies, that breed may not work for another person's.

For that reason, I always recommend getting to know the breed first to make sure there is no reaction.

2. Myths about Hypoallergenic

When it comes to myths regarding hypoallergenic dogs, there are a lot of them. Let's face it; people want to own a dog and it is very easy to create a myth or be told one. Before you commit to a hypoallergenic dog, it is important to understand what the myths about hypoallergenic dogs are so you can be aware of what the truth is surrounding them.

Myth: People are only allergic to the fur.

Fact:

While the fur may seem like the actual reason behind a person's allergies, it is not the only reason. As I have mentioned already, dogs produce a protein, and it is this protein that causes the allergic reaction.

This protein is found on the fur, or more specifically the hair root, saliva, dander (skin cells, similar to dandruff in humans), and also in the dog's urine. So while we may have less chances of coming into contact with the saliva or urine, it can still be a trigger for someone who has allergies.

Myth: Hairless dogs are always hypoallergenic.

Fact:

While many people who suffer from allergies find they are able to breathe easier with hairless dogs, it is not a sure-fire way to have a hypoallergenic dog. Remember, it all goes back to the dander and oils found on the skin. Hairless dogs still have these oils so they can create allergic reactions just as easily as a dog with a long coat.

Myth: If I am allergic to one type of dog, I am allergic to them all.

Fact:

While having allergies to dogs can mean being allergic to a large number of them, many people who suffer from allergies find that certain dog breeds, and coats, do not bother their allergies as much as others.

Myth: Allergy sufferers can only own small-sized dogs.

Fact:

There have been studies that suggest that smaller dogs are a better choice for allergy sufferers, but they aren't the only choice. While small dogs produce smaller amounts of the allergen due to their size, there are many larger breeds that also produce smaller amounts.

For that reason, you can have a range of sizes to choose from when you are choosing your dog. Later in this book, I will go through some of the most popular hypoallergenic dog breed choices that range from the tiny Yorkshire Terrier to the large Samoyed.

Myth: There really are 100% hypoallergenic dogs.

Fact:

No dog is completely hypoallergenic. While they may not produce as much of the allergen as other breeds, they still produce it. It is important to keep this in mind when choosing to get a dog.

Myth: All designer breeds with Poodle in the cross are hypoallergenic.

Fact:

One interesting fact about designer breeds, such as the Labradoodle, is that they all started because of one breeder in Australia. In an effort to create a hypoallergenic service dog to work with patients who have allergies, the Labradoodle was created. His goal was to produce a dog with the temperament of a Labrador Retriever with the coat of a Poodle, the latter of which had been proven to have fewer allergens.

The result was the Labradoodle, and the age of designer breeds quickly took off from there. Unfortunately, the Labradoodle was a failed experiment, and while the breed is wonderful in and of itself, it was quickly realized that they weren't as hypoallergenic as expected.

The reason for this, which can be applied to any Poodle cross, is that only one coat type seems to produce that hypoallergenic effect -- the curly/wavy coat. The remaining coats can produce the same allergic reaction as the average dog.

Myth: If you have allergies, you will always have allergies.

Fact:

Although avoidance is often the best choice when you have an allergy, there are people who can live with dogs even when they are allergic to them. The reason for this is because immunity to the dog dander will build over time.

So while the allergy doesn't go away, per se, it does become reduced enough where you can be around dogs without having an allergic reaction.

In addition, studies have shown that early exposure to dog dander can reduce the chance of developing allergies. This is excellent in regards to kids. Children who grow up with dogs are less likely to be allergic to them.

Myth: If I have allergies, I can't own a dog.

Fact:

This goes hand in hand with the last myth, but having allergies does not keep you from owning a dog. In fact, you can own one of the many hypoallergenic breeds listed in this book.

Also, if you follow the helpful tips to reducing canine allergens in your home, you can live a very happy life with a dog.

Myth: Dogs with hair-like coats are more hypoallergenic than those with fur.

Fact:

While some people find the hair-like coats to be easier to handle when it comes to allergies, this is not always the case. Remember that it is the protein, found on the skin and in the dander, that affects allergy sufferers. So if a dog produces a lot of the protein, it won't matter what type of coat it has.

As you can see, there are a lot of myths, but the facts are with proper management, choosing the right breed, and being aware of your own limitations in regards to your allergies, you can live with a dog.

3. What Makes a Dog Hypoallergenic?

As you know, there is no such thing as a truly hypoallergenic dog. So when we sit down and list traits of a dog, it is really not a foolproof option.

However, that being said, there are still points that you should look for in a dog, which can help determine if the breed has hypoallergenic qualities or not.

One: Non-Shedding Breeds

Yes, I did say that fur is not the only contributor to allergens; however, the protein that is the cause of allergies usually clings to the hair. Dogs that shed leave fewer allergens in their environment. So breeds with wire coats, curly coats, and hairless coats are less likely to deposit allergens than those who have shedding coats.

Two: Smaller Breeds

Yes, there are some larger breeds that are hypoallergenic; however, studies have shown that smaller breeds are less likely to spread dander in their environment.

Less dander means less of the allergen. It has been proven that smaller dogs leave less of an impact in their environment, and this makes it much easier for allergy sufferers to breathe easy around them.

Three: Length of Coat

This does not apply to everyone, but many allergy sufferers have a harder time when a dog has a longer coat. It is the added fur that can lead to the increase in allergens being released in the home. In addition, fur often acts as a secondary trigger for allergies, so the longer hair can lead to more allergy attacks.

On the other side, some people suffer more with really short coats. The reason for this is because the protein is easily accessible in short-haired dogs. If the dog produces the regular amount or more dander than other dogs, they are more likely to trigger the allergic reaction.

Four: Indoor Breeds

Breeds that are better suited to indoors are often more likely to be hypoallergenic. Outdoor dogs, or breeds that spend a lot of time outside, often pick up molds, pollen, and other allergens that can trigger allergic reactions.

Actually, dogs that spend more time inside than outside are less likely to create allergy problems than those who spend a large amount of their time outside.

Five: Clean Breeds

Yes, there can be clean dog breeds, and this usually refers to breeds that don't shed, don't drool, and are less likely to bring in dirt and mud on their paws. Avoid breeds that drool (eg. Mastiffs), as well as breeds that bring in dirt and allergens (eg. Newfoundlands). Other breeds to avoid are ones that shed (eg. Labrador Retrievers). All of these breeds are a poor fit for allergy sufferers and should be avoided.

So when you are choosing a dog breed, make sure you research it to find out if it is a messier breed.

And those are the traits that you should look for in your hypoallergenic breeds. In the next chapter, I have included a list of hypoallergenic breeds where you can begin your research.

Chapter Two: Choosing the Right Hypoallergenic Breed

Now that you understand the myths about hypoallergenic dog breeds, it is time to go over a few tips with finding the right breed for you. Even with allergies, there is a right breed and there is a wrong breed, and making the wrong choice can make life with your dog miserable.

In the last chapter, I looked at what traits to look for in a hypoallergenic breed. In this chapter, we will be covering what to look for in a hypoallergenic dog breeder and the breed of the individual puppy you are purchasing to match your lifestyle.

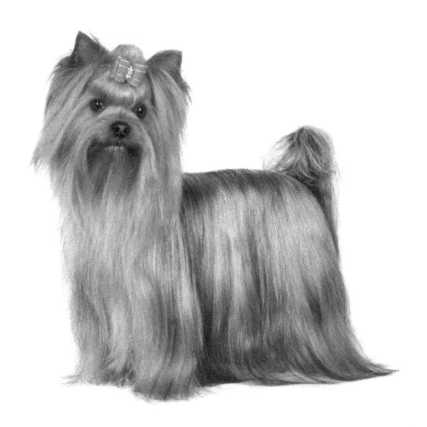

1. What to Look For

When it comes to looking for a dog, it is important to do it properly. Never purchase a dog on a whim when the mood hits you. Remember, trying to choose a hypoallergenic breed and buying on a whim can lead to you choosing a breed that isn't hypoallergenic.

Next, it is important to research the breeds and then research the breeders. If you fail to research, you could purchase from lines that have serious health problems. While this won't affect whether the dog is hypoallergenic or not, it could lead to heartbreak and very expensive vet bills for you.

Some tips that you should follow when you are looking for a puppy are as follows:

Tip Number One: Research Where You Are Buying

First, when you are ready to bring a puppy home, take the time to research where you are going to be purchasing from. There are many different ways to get a dog, and all of them have different guidelines.

Registered Breeder:

One place that many people purchase their puppy from is a registered breeder. It is very important that you do your research to make sure you are purchasing a puppy from an ethical breeder.

If you choose a breeder, ask to see health clearances for the dogs. Also ask if they compete in showing or some other activity with their dogs. A dog that spends 80% of its life in a kennel is not ideal, and you should avoid breeders who do this. Kennelling is not a problem exactly, but the dogs should also spend time out of the kennel.

Another thing to look at with registered breeders is the cleanliness of their facility. Always go and visit the breeder so you can view their facilities. Puppies should be raised indoors with plenty of socialization. The puppy room, kennels, and overall home should be clean. If it isn't, or the dogs are kept in cramp quarters, find a different breeder.

One rule that I have for anyone who is purchasing from a breeder is to go with their gut feeling. If, at any time, you have a bad feeling about the breeder, find a new one.

Also, expect a waiting list. Reputable breeders often have a waiting list before you can purchase a puppy. If you find an excellent breeder, go on the waiting list; trust me, you won't be disappointed.

Rescue Groups and Shelters

Many people ignore rescue groups when they are looking for a puppy because they believe that they can only adopt adult dogs from them. While there is a need for people to adopt older dogs, it is not uncommon for rescue groups to have puppies or pregnant females.

In addition, mixed breeds are very common, especially when you are looking for a designer dog, but there are also many purebred dogs in rescues and shelters.

With rescue groups, follow the same advice as I gave you with breeders. Always visit the rescue group and do plenty of research on them. While there are hundreds of exceptional rescue groups out there, there are also many that are subpar and the dogs are poorly treated.

When you go and visit a rescue, make sure that all the dogs look like they are being cared for. You may see dogs in various stages of health due to them being rescued from bad conditions, but the dogs that are available for adoption should be healthy. Also, the facilities should be clean.

If the dogs are fostered, find out as much as you can about the rescue and the fosters. They should be as picky about you as you are about them.

Make sure all the puppies or dogs are up to date on vaccinations and that the rescue group is open about the dog's past and treatment since being in the shelter or rescue group. Remember that if the dog was picked up as a stray, they may not have a lot of information about its past before ending up in a shelter.

Individuals

If you are looking for an older dog, you can always adopt an older dog from an owner. Be aware that there are a lot of reasons why people will get rid of their dogs, and many times, it is because of behavioral problems.

While I do not recommend avoiding personal ads for dogs, remember that you may have to deal with some problems you weren't expecting.

Always plan to take the dog to a vet for a check-up, even if the person says it has been checked. Also take the dog to a behaviorist or dog trainer. Again, this will help correct any issues earlier than if you try on your own.

If you can, try to get the medical history of the dog and find out what its life has been like up until that point. Has it been rehomed before? Has it had any surgeries? Is it intact or has it been neutered or spayed?

Finding out as much as you can about the dog before you rehome it, can help the dog better adjust to your home.

When it comes to buying, never purchase a dog from a puppy mill or a store. Stores often purchase their puppies from puppy mills, and puppy mills often keep their puppies in filthy, cramped conditions. Puppies are usually ill, and the parents of the puppies are even worse.

Puppy mills breed for money and put very little care into their puppies. Saving a puppy from a mill without the mill being shut down only keeps the puppy mill going since it is making money.

Another place to be aware of is a puppy broker or puppy flipper. These are people who purchase a puppy and then resell it for more than they initially paid. Or they purchase puppies from places outside the country where there aren't many restrictions.

Puppy brokers often take the puppies at a too young age, and all of the dogs are kept in poor conditions until they are sold.

Tip Number Two: Always Ask Questions

Regardless of where you are purchasing your puppy, you should have a list of questions that you ask the breeder or shelter. Some common questions to ask breeders are:

1. Have any of the puppies from the litter been sick?
2. Have any of your dogs had an inherent disease?
3. Are the puppies sold with first vaccinations?
4. Are the puppies dewormed?
5. Do you do any dog activities with your dogs?
6. How are the parents in regards to temperament and health?
7. Are the puppies raised in the home?
8. Are the puppies socialized?
9. What is the history of the parents and grandparents?
10. Is there a health certificate or guarantee sold with the puppies?

Common questions to ask the shelter or rescue:

1. What condition was the dog found in?
2. Was it an owner surrender, found as a stray, or from an abusive situation?
3. Has it had any behavioral issues? If so, what, and have they been addressed?
4. Is the dog neutered or spayed?
5. What vaccinations and health care has it received?
6. Has it been temperament tested with cats, dogs, and people?
7. Has it been rehomed before? If so, why was it brought back to the rescue?
8. Do you offer any support for your new owners?
9. How long has it been in the shelter?
10. Has it been to foster homes? If so, how many?

Make sure that you always take the time to get your answers. If the breeder or group does not want to answer your questions, choose a different one.

Tip Number Three: Visit

Always take the time to visit the breeder or shelter at least one time before you go and pick up your puppy. The reason for this is you are more likely to see problems if you have gone to the location several times.

Look around, and if you find that the location is dirty or the dogs appear unhealthy or scared, choose a different breeder. Purchasing a puppy from a dirty place could lead to many health problems down the road. It also shows that the breeder may not be putting much effort into the care of the puppies, which could lead to behavioral problems later on.

Tip Number Four: Check the Health of your Puppy

Whenever you go to look at a puppy, always check the health of your puppy. What this means is that you need to do a quick health check of not just the puppy you are interested in getting but in all of the puppies. While there can be a sick puppy in a litter, if the breeder will not explain the illness or more than one puppy is sick, you may want to avoid purchasing from that litter.

To do a health check, you want to start by looking at all the puppies. Are they playing? Do they look alert and hydrated? If the puppies look flat when they are sleeping, sort of listless, then something may be wrong. If they all seem fine, start doing a head to tail tip examination while you play with them.

Always start by examining the head. You should see the following traits:

- *Nose:* The nose should be moist when you touch it. Also, there should be a cool feel to it. There should never be discharge, and while one or two sneezes are fine, a puppy that is sneezing frequently may be sick.

- *Teeth:* Get the puppy to close its mouth, and look at its teeth. Are any broken? Are the gums bleeding? What is the bite like? This will differ depending on the breed, but most breeds need a scissor-like bite. This is when the top teeth slightly overlap the lower teeth. An uneven bite can signify a problem, but many times it is just cosmetic.

- *Gums:* While you are looking at the teeth, make sure the gums are pink. If they are pale, there could be a parasite or another health problem.

- *Eyes:* Eyes should be bright and free of any mucus or discharge. They should be clear, and you should be able to see the haw, which is a third eyelid. The eyes should not be swollen, and if you see white spots or lines in the pupils, it could signify an eye problem later in life.

- *Ears:* Ears should be alert and held properly for the breed. There should be no dirt in the ears, and they should have a sweet smell to them.

Once you are done looking at the head, move down the body. Run your hand over the puppy and feel for anything strange. Check the fur for flea dander or fleas and also look for bare spots or crusty spots on the puppy. This could be mange.

Pick the puppy up and feel its breathing. It should be an even in and out, and you can feel when there is trouble breathing. Also, feel the heart. It should be fast and clear.

Finally, always touch the dome of the skull. If there is a soft spot, you want to avoid that puppy. Many toy breeds can suffer from an open fontanel, and it can indicate a condition called hydrocephalus, which is where there is an abnormal amount of fluid in the brain.

Tip Number Five: Listen to the Breeder

Finally, when you are searching for your puppy, it is important to listen to your breeder in regards to picks. Some breeders will make the choice for you, but even those who don't, it is important to listen to them.

The main reason for this is because the breeder has been with the puppies for eight weeks. They know which ones are more dominant and which ones are not as hyper. They will know the shy ones and the outgoing pups, and they will be able to help match the perfect pup to your lifestyle.

In the end, however, you have to be happy with your puppy, so if, at any time, you feel like the match is not working, walk away from the purchase. Trust me; if you do, both you and the puppy will be happier.

2. Finding the Right Breed for Your Lifestyle

Although I already went through what to look for when you are purchasing a puppy, before you begin your search, it is very important to research dog breeds so you can find the best breed for you.

In the next section, I have compiled a list of hypoallergenic breeds, and the list is a great basis to get started on selecting a breed. Before you do the research, however, it is important to ask yourself a few questions:

How much time do I have for a puppy?

All breeds require a lot of time as puppies; however, when they get older, some breeds are independent and don't need to spend as much time with their owners as others. Other breeds suffer significantly when their owners are away, and this can lead to behavioral problems.

Even still, you will need to have a few hours of dedicated time for your dog every day. These hours take into account playtime, walks, training, and simply showing affection to your dog. If you work long hours and will constantly be away, having a puppy or dog may not be the best fit for you, regardless of allergies.

Am I active?

If you love going for hikes, getting outdoors, or doing a sport that your dog can be involved in, then choose an active breed such as a Boxerdoodle or a Portuguese Water Dog. If you prefer to curl up on the couch with a good book, choose a companion breed with low energy such as a Shih Tzu.

If you enjoy a blend of both active hobbies and curling up at home, choose a dog with a medium energy level such as a Bichon Frise or a Newfypoo.

This is a very important thing to consider as choosing the wrong energy level for your lifestyle can make owning a dog more of a chore and less of an enjoyment.

Where do I live?

You are in luck when it comes to hypoallergenic breeds since most of the breeds can do well in any location. However, there are a few breeds that should not be in apartments and do much better in the countryside. Komodors are one breed where they need room to roam.

In addition, some breeds can be quite loud, such as the Yorkshire Terrier, so if you live in an apartment with a noise restriction, the breed may not be the right breed for you.

In general, smaller dog breeds are better suited to apartment living, but larger, low energy dogs can do well in them too. In addition, energy level can affect where you live. While a medium-sized dog may fit in an apartment, high energy level breeds, such as the Aussiedoodle, are better suited to homes with a fenced yard.

Have I owned a dog before?

Another question to answer is whether you have owned a dog before. This should be a dog on your own, not a family dog as a child. If you haven't, I recommend that you choose a breed that doesn't have as much maintenance requirements as others.

In addition, I recommend that you choose breeds that are eager to please and are known for being easy to train. Choosing a stubborn breed, such as a Mastidoodle, can make owning that first dog challenging.

If you have owned a dog before, then there really is no limit as long as you are willing to put in the time to train the dog properly.

What is my patience level with grooming?

Many of the hypoallergenic breeds have few grooming needs; however, some can require quite a lot of grooming. Every dog needs general grooming such as teeth cleaning, nail trimming, and bathing, so be aware of how much grooming you can enjoy doing.

If you decide you want to hire a groomer for your dog, remember that the harder the coat is to care for, the higher the cost will be for you.

What is my budget?

Finally, be honest about your budget and not just for the purchase price of the puppy. Remember that the puppy will cost you anywhere from a few hundred to a few thousand dollars to purchase.

In addition, once the puppy comes home, you will have several hundred dollars in vet bills. In fact, that first year of life usually costs around US$1500 (£900 or €1100) and then US$500 to $600 (£300 to £360 or €375 to €450) per year after that.

Often, larger breeds cost more, and if your breed has health problems, the overall lifetime expenses could be significantly more. If you have a smaller budget, you should be looking at a healthier, smaller dog breed.

Once you have answered those questions, it is time to look at the different breeds that match your needs. Start by selecting ten breeds that you love the look of. When you have those ten breeds, read up on each one.

Cross off breeds that you know won't fit into your lifestyle. Be honest and don't try to make them fit or you and the dog will be very unhappy.

After you have crossed off some breeds, do more research and try to meet as many of those breeds as possible. Go to dog shows, dog parks, or any other canine event. You want to meet adult dogs since all puppies are cute, and it is very easy to fall in love with them. However, that puppy does grow up, and the adult dog can be very different.

Try to narrow down that list to three breeds that you are really interested in. Now is the time to start researching breeders. Start with breeders in your immediate area and ask to go visit the breed. Meet the adults at the kennel and find ways to meet other adult dogs. Again, this helps you decide if it is the right dog for you.

Join breed groups, forums, or clubs to get a better understanding of the breeds you are interested in. Trust me; once you have had time with your top three breeds, you will quickly realize which breed is the best for you and your family.

After that, it is as simple as selecting the top one out of those three breeds and then making plans to bring your puppy home, which we went over in the last section.

3. List of Hypoallergenic Dog Breeds

When it comes to hypoallergenic dog breeds, there are actually several dozen breeds that have a low level of allergens on their skin. This low level makes them the perfect choice for people who have allergies. While I would love to go into detail of every breed, this book focuses on the top 15 dog breeds for allergy sufferers. However, I do want you to be aware of all the possibilities regarding dog breeds so I have created a list of hypoallergenic breeds in a small chart, which lists the breed, their size, and their energy levels.

Dog Breed	Size	Energy Level
Afghan Hound	Large	Medium
Affenpoo	Toy	High
Airedale Terrier	Medium	Very High
Airedoodle	Medium to Large	Very High
American Hairless Terrier	Toy	High
Aussiedoodle	Medium	High to Very High
Australian Terrier	Toy	High
Barbet	Medium	High
Basenji	Medium	High
Bassetoodle	Medium	Low to Medium
Bedlington Terrier	Small	Medium
Bergamasco	Medium	High
Bernedoodle	Large	Medium to High
Bichon Frise	Toy	Medium
Bichon Yorkie	Toy	Medium to High
Bich-Poo	Toy to Small	Medium
Bolodoodle	Toy to Small	High
Bolognese	Toy	High
Border Terrier	Small	High
Bordoodle	Medium to Large	Very High
Bossi-Poo	Small	High
Bouvier des Flanders	Large	High
Boxerdoodle	Medium to Large	Very High
Broodle Griffon	Toy	Medium
Brussels Griffon	Toy	Medium
Bull Terrier	Small	High
Ca-doodle	Small to Large	Medium to High
Cairnoodle	Toy to Small	High
Cairn Terrier	Toy	High
Cavachon	Small	Medium
Cavapoo	Small	Medium to High
Cesky Terrier	Small	Medium
Chacy Ranior	Small	High
Chinese Crested	Toy	Low

Chinese Crestpoo	Toy to Small	Low to Medium
Chipoo	Toy to Small	Medium
Cockapoo	Small	Medium
Corgipoo	Small	Medium
Coton De Tulear	Toy	Medium
Daisy Dog	Toy	Medium
Dalmadoodle	Large	Very High
Dandie Dinmont Terrier	Small	Medium
Doodleman Pinscher	Medium to Large	High
Double Doodle	Large	High
Doxiepoo	Small	Medium to High
English Boodle	Medium	Low
Eskipoo	Toy, Small and Medium	High
Flandoodle	Large	Very High
Foodle	Small	High
Foxhoodle	Medium	High
Goldendoodle	Large	High
Great Danoodle	Large to Giant	High to Very High
Hairless Khala	Toy to Small	Medium
Havanese	Toy	Low
Irish Doodle	Medium to Large	Very High
Irish Terrier	Small	High
Irish Troodle	Small	High
Irish Water Spaniel	Medium	Very High
Italian Greyhound	Small	Medium
Jack-a-Poo	Small	Very High
Kerry Blue Terrier	Medium	High
Komondor	Large	Medium to High
Labradoodle	Large	High
Lacasapoo	Toy to Small	Low to Medium
Lagotta Romagnolo	Medium	High
Lhasapoo	Toy to Small	Low
Lakeland Terrier	Small	High
Lowchen	Small	Medium
Maltese	Toy	Medium
Malti-Poo	Toy to Small	Medium to High

Mastidoodle	Large to Giant	Low
Miniature Aussiedoodle	Small	Very High
Native American Indian Dog	Medium to Large	Medium
Newfypoo	Large to Giant	Medium
Norfolk Terrier	Toy	High
Norwich Terrier	Toy	High
Papipoo	Toy	Medium
Pekepoo	Toy	Medium
Peruvian Inca Orchid	Medium	Medium
Pinny-Poo	Toy	High
Polish Lowland Sheepdog	Medium	High
Pomapoo	Toy	Medium
Poo-Shi	Small	High
Poo-Ton	Toy to Small	Medium
Poochin	Toy	Medium
Poodle	Toy, Small and Large	High
Poogle	Small	Very High
Poolky	Toy	High
Pootalian	Toy	Medium
Poovanese	Toy to Small	Low
Portuguese Water Dog	Medium	Very High
Pugapoo	Small	Medium to High
Puli	Medium	High
Pyredoodle	Large to Giant	Medium to High
Rattle	Small	High
Rottle	Large	Medium to High
Saint Berdoodle	Large to Giant	Medium
Samoyed	Medium	Medium
Schipper-Poo	Small	High
Schnauzer	Small, Medium and Large	High to Very High
Schnoodle	Small, Medium and Large	High to Very High
Scoodle	Small	High

Scottish Terrier	Toy	High
Sealyham Terrier	Small	Medium
Sheltidoodle	Large	High
Sheepadoodle	Large	High
Shepadoodle	Large	High
Shichon	Small	High
Shih-Poo	Toy	Low
Shih Tzu	Toy	Low
Siberpoo	Medium to Large	High to Very High
Silky Terrier	Toy	High
Skypoo	Toy to Small	High
Soft Coated Wheaten Terrier	Medium	High
Spanish Water Dog	Medium	High
Springerdoodle	Small to Medium	Very High
Terri-Poo	Toy	High
Tibetan Terrier	Medium	High
Ttoodle	Small	Medium
Weimardoodle	Large	Very High
Welsh Terrier	Small	High
West Highland White Terrier	Small	Medium
Westiepoo	Small	Medium
Whoodle	Medium	High
Wire Fox Terrier	Small	High
Wire-haired Pointing Griffon	Medium	High
Wire-Poo	Small	High
Woodle	Small	High
Xoloitzcuintle	Toy, Small and Medium	Medium
Yorkipoo	Toy	Medium
Yorkshire Terrier	Toy	Low

Chapter Three: Fighting Allergens

So you found the perfect breed for you and your family. That is terrific, but finding a hypoallergenic dog is not the last step to making sure that your allergies are managed.

As I have said, there is no such thing as a 100% hypoallergenic dog. They can come very close, but there are still things you will need to do to help keep your allergies at bay. In this chapter, I will go over the best ways to manage your allergies and how to reduce those allergens in your home.

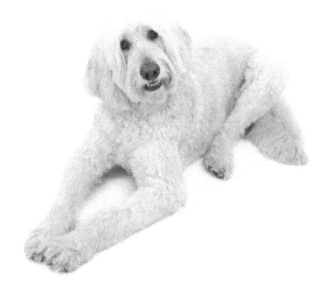

1. Tips for Managing Allergies with a Dog

While most allergy experts will all agree that the best way to manage your allergies is to not own a dog, it is not always practical advice. For many dog lovers, the flare up of allergies is worth the time spent with their beloved pooch.

However, it doesn't have to be that way, and starting with a hypoallergenic pet is the first step to ensuring you can own a dog. In addition to the breed, it is important to follow a number of tips that will make living with a dog much easier for your sinuses.

Tip Number One: Keep Dogs Off the Furniture

First, try to keep your pets off of the furniture. This will help cut down on the dander on places where you are sitting. Dander on furniture, especially fabrics, is difficult to get off, and you will often be overwhelmed by the allergens.

Tip Number Two: Make Designated Dog Rooms

Another tip is to make sure the dog has set rooms in the home to give you a place to escape to when you are having a bad day. These dog-free zones will have less dander in them and can make managing your allergies much easier.

Tip Number Three: Make Your Bedroom A Dog-Free Room

This goes hand in hand with tip number two, but many people don't think about making their bedrooms dog-free. They often allow the dog into the bedroom at night and can't figure out why their allergies are triggered in the morning.

Even if the allergies are not triggered, often allowing the dog to sleep in your room can lead to restless sleep, migraines, and other problems. It can leave you feeling unwell with no real reason for it.

Keeping the dog out of the room will help with this and will keep you happy and breathing easy.

One common rule I have in the house is the dog is not allowed upstairs where the bedrooms are. This keeps hair to a minimum upstairs and ensures that everyone in the house sleeps easy.

Tip Number Four: Have Tile or Hardwood

This isn't possible for everyone, but have tiled or hardwood flooring. Carpet traps the allergens and makes it very difficult to manage your allergies.

If you can't replace the carpet in your home, purchase a good vacuum, such as a Dyson Animal or similar model. Using a subpar vacuum will keep the allergens in the carpet and you can release them into the air.

Tip Number Five: Give Your Dog an Outside Area

A screened-in porch or a balcony for the dog to relax in is a perfect way to help manage your allergies since the dog will not be depositing all of the allergens inside.

By following these tips, you should be able to manage your allergies. If you do have a reaction, try to avoid taking an allergy medication unless it is absolutely necessary. If you do take them too often, you can create an immunity to the allergy medication and not to the allergen.

Instead, allow your body to build up a tolerance to the allergen, and over time, the allergic reactions will begin to decrease.

2. Reducing Allergens in your Home

While the tips that I have given you when it comes to managing your allergies will help in reducing the allergens in your home, there are several things that you can do in addition to managing your home and allergies.

One: Bathe Your Dog Frequently

First, it is important to bathe your dog frequently at the body temperature of the dog (no hotter). This will help reduce the amount of allergen that builds up on the dog's skin and coat.

Although there are different recommendations regarding bathing and coat type, when you are trying to reduce the allergens in your home, it is important to wash your dog on a weekly basis.

Two: Brush Daily

Before you follow this tip, make sure you understand the coat type of your dog. Some coat types, such as the wiry coat of the Airedale Terrier, should not be brushed. Instead, you would need to strip the coat, which is only done once or twice a year.

Three: Clean the House Frequently

Make a weekly schedule to clean your house to remove allergens. Generally, allergens hide on the floor, on the top of tables and furniture, and on windowsills. You should also clean on the top of doors and around window frames.

Cleaning your home should be easy, and usually just a damp cloth is enough to remove the allergies.

When you clean, wear a mask if you have severe allergies, as cleaning will kick up the allergens into the air.

Four: Use a HEPA Filter

You can purchase a HEPA air purifier, and you can also purchase vacuum cleaners with HEPA filters. This helps remove particles from the air and will greatly reduce the number of allergens in your home.

Five: Keep Your House Cool

Another important tip for reducing the number of allergens in your home, including pet allergens, is to keep your home cool. Try to maintain a temperature of between 68 to 72°F (20-22°C).

In addition, try to keep your home at 50% humidity or lower. High temperatures and humidity usually increase the number of dust mites in the house and also the amount of mold.

While you may not have an allergy to dust or mold, the increase of both can aggravate your allergies.

Tip Number Seven: Clean Your Filters Monthly

Make a habit of cleaning your heating and ventilation filters monthly. Dog hair and dander often get sucked into your ventilation system, and this will aggravate your allergies.

Changing the filters monthly will help reduce the amount of allergens in your home.

Tip Number Eight: Wash Drapes and Curtains Monthly

Every month, wash the curtains and drapes in your home with hot water. If you can, use color-safe bleach when you are washing them to help kill any mite or other allergen that is in the curtains.

Dry them completely before you hang them back up to prevent cross contaminating them with new dander and hair.

Tip Number Nine: Close the Registers

If you have forced air, you can reduce the amount of allergens in your home simply by closing the registers. This will keep the hair and dander out of the ventilation system as much as possible and you are less likely to suffer from allergic reactions.

If you find that it is impossible to close the registers, try closing the registers in the rooms where your dog is.

Tip Number Ten: Groom Outside

Finally, when you are grooming your dog, always groom it outside, even with bathing. When a dog is washed, the warm water often loosens up the hair and you end up with a lot in the home.

This also releases a large amount of the protein into the environment, and you have a greater risk of having an allergic reaction at this time.

If you can, take them to a groomer so you won't risk a reaction.

And those are all the tips I can give you for managing your allergies and reducing the allergens in your home. But again, it all starts with choosing the perfect, hypoallergenic breed.

Chapter Four: Top 10 Hypoallergenic Purebreds

While understanding how to reduce allergens will greatly increase the enjoyment you have with your dog, choosing the right breed is central to this enjoyment. Trust me; choosing the wrong breed will only lead you to feel frustrated with the dog, and in the end, it will be a failed relationship.

Although I would love to go through all of the different, hypoallergenic breeds you can choose, I felt it would be overwhelming. Instead, I want to focus on a select few breeds to give you the foundation.

In this chapter, I will be going over the top ten purebred breeds that you can choose from. This is only a handful, but they are the most popular, hypoallergenic breeds out there.

I will take you through each breed, the size, temperament, and history of the breed, as well as the health problems that each breed has. I will also take you through the pros and cons of the breed and all the other information you will need.

By the end of each breed profile, you should have a clear understanding of the breed and whether it will fit into your home and lifestyle.

This chapter is on purebred breeds. A purebred dog is a dog that has been bred from parents of the exact same breed. In addition, their parents were also bred from parents of the exact same breed of dog. So let's get started with the first breed.

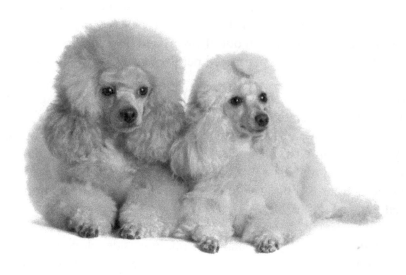

1. The Intelligent Poodle

They are known as being a breed that is all about looks, but did you know the Poodle was originally designed for function? They were, in fact, designed to be a hunting dog, and while they are not commonly used in that capacity today, they still have the drive you see in working breeds.

But where other working breeds have a set size, the Poodle can be found in several sizes, which makes it an ideal breed for any allergy sufferer, regardless of living conditions. In addition, the coat of the Poodle is believed to be the best hypoallergenic coat, which is why it has gone into making so many doodle breeds.

a) History of the Breed

One interesting fact about the Poodle is that while it is closely linked to France, the breed was developed in Germany. In fact, the purpose of the Poodle was for it to be a waterfowl birding dog.

It was believed that the curly coat of the Poodle would give it better protection from the elements and landscape, particularly when it was entering water. However, over the years, the primary use of the breed has fallen out of favor, and now the Poodle spends more time as a pampered pet than a rugged hunting dog.

While we know what it was originally developed for, it is unclear what breed went into developing the Poodle. It is believed that the breed can be dated back to Asian herding dogs that were adopted by the Germanic Goth and Ostrogoth tribes. It is also speculated that the breed may date back as early as Ancient Egypt since there are depictions of Poodle-like dogs on tombs and artifacts from that era.

Many enthusiasts believe that the Poodle was developed by crossing the North African Barbet with the Spanish Water Dog as well as with the German Water Dog, Russian Water Dog, Hungarian Water Dog, Portuguese Water Dog, and the French Water Dog.

The first was documented before the 1400s and is considered to be one of the oldest hunting breeds. The first Poodle was the larger, Standard Poodle; however, when the breed became popular in France, breeders began creating smaller Poodles.

In fact, by the 1400s, both the toy and miniature Poodle were established and were quite popular with the Parisian bourgeoise. Even in those days, the Poodle was still being used as a hunting dog, while the Miniature Poodle was used to find truffles and the Toy Poodle was a lap dog. All of the Poodle varieties were used as circus dogs since their intelligence made them perfect dogs for the work.

The breed was first recognized by the Kennel Club of England in 1874 and by the American Kennel Club in 1886. The breed club was established in 1896, disbanded and reformed in 1931.

While the popularity of the Poodle waned for many years, today it is one of the most popular dog breeds and is a top choice for people with allergies.

b) Temperament of the Breed

If you are looking for an intelligent companion that is loving and attentive, then look no further than a Poodle. This is a breed that is known for its playful personality and mischievous temperament. They often get into things, but their goofy playfulness keeps them from getting into trouble for it.

They are usually quick to train; however, they can be a bit timid and shy, which can make training a bit difficult. The Poodle is usually reserved with strangers and can often be fearful of them if they are not properly socialized.

The breed is known for having a dignified air about them, and they are definitely a noble breed. They do enjoy barking and can become problem barking if they are allowed. They are alert and can make an excellent watch dog, although their timid nature makes them unsuitable for guarding.

c) Appearance of the Breed

The Poodle is a small- to large-sized dog that is known for its curly coat and interesting hairstyles. However, that is not all that makes up the Poodle. They should have a square appearance with the length of the dog being equal to the height at the shoulders. The top line of the dog should be level and straight.

Poodles should have a head that is refined with a moderately round skull and a long, straight muzzle. The muzzle should have a definite stop. Eyes should be oval shaped and should be set slightly far apart. They should be dark and either black or brown in color.

Ears of the Poodle should be long and hanging. They should be kept close to the head. They should never be carried high and should never be cropped. The tail should be medium in length and carried high.

The breed should be graceful and elegant. In general, females are smaller than males; however, it is often difficult to tell the difference between the two as they have very similar features.

i. Coat

The Poodle should have a thick double coat, with a curly or corded texture. The color of the Poodle can be any solid color. They can also be parti-colored, which is one color with white; however, it is not allowed in show Poodles. Common colors that you see in Poodles are red, brown, silver, black, white, blue, cream, cafe-au-lait, or apricot.

ii. Size

As I have mentioned, there are three sizes for Poodles, although they all have the same structure and coat. These are:

Toy:
>   Up to 10 inches (25.4cm) in height
>   6 to 9 pounds (2.72 to 4.1kg) in weight

Miniature:
>   11 to 15 inches (27.9 to 38.1cm) in height
>   15 to 17 pounds (16.8 to 7.7kg) in weight

Standard:
>   15 to 22 inches (38.1 to 55.9cm) or more in height
>   45 to 70 pounds (20.1 to 31.8kg) in weight

d) The Needs of the Breed

Poodles, like all breeds, have specific needs that should be taken care of on a daily basis. This includes grooming, exercise, and training. Before you purchase a Poodle, make sure you understand the needs of the breed.

i. Exercise

The Poodle is an active breed with a lot of energy, so they need to be exercised. In general, most Poodles need to be walked several times a day or up to about an hour a day. They love to do activities and should be given time to run off leash in a secure area.

In addition to physical exercise, you should give your Poodle plenty of intellectual exercise. Give them problem solving toys to keep them from becoming bored. A bored Poodle will find ways to amuse itself, and they can become destructive.

Another important exercise is daily training. Even as an adult, you should train your Poodle about once a day for ten to fifteen minutes a day.

ii. Living Conditions

As I mentioned earlier, the Poodle can fit into any type of living condition. They are generally quiet and calm inside, which is why they can do well in apartments.

Even the Standard Poodle, which is the largest, can do well in an apartment. It is good for the Poodle to have some access to outside and can do well in homes with a small yard.

iii. Ease of Training

When it comes to training, the Poodle is a very intelligent breed that can learn very quickly. That being said, it is important to remember that sometimes intelligence can make them stubborn. They often have a mind of their own, and if they become bored with training, they will begin to act up.

In addition to this natural stubbornness, the Poodle can be shy and timid. This makes it very important to use positive reinforcement for training instead of correction. Any harsh corrections can have lifelong effects on your dog's temperament, so it should be avoided with the Poodle.

Another factor that should be taken into account with the Poodle is the shy temperament. It is imperative that you socialize your Poodle at a young age so the puppy does not grow fearful or aggressive toward strangers. Make sure that you also socialize your pup with other dogs and animals.

Finally, with the smaller varieties of the Poodle, don't be tempted with carrying it around or treating it like a human. Toy and miniature Poodles can be prone to Small Dog Syndrome, which will lead to problem barking, destructive behavior, and even aggression.

iv. Grooming Requirements

There are two different sides to the grooming requirements of a Poodle. On one hand, if you choose to keep the coat short, the care is quite easy. You can take the dog to a groomer and have its coat shaved down to a cut that is known as a puppy coat.

With this cut, bathing can be kept at a minimum; however, I still recommend once a week for allergies, and the dog can be brushed only when necessary or at the time of the clipping. The coat should be clipped every three to six weeks to keep it short.

If you are opting for a full coat or for a styled coat, you will have more work to deal with. The coat will need daily brushing, and you will need to trim it frequently to keep the style looking fresh. Bathing will need to be done weekly.

In addition to bathing and brushing, you will need to clean the ears weekly. The nails will also need to be trimmed at least once per month, and you should trim the hair around footpads.

Finally, on lighter colored Poodles, you will need to wash around the eyes as it is very common for the area to become stained by tears.

e) Health of the Breed

The average lifespan of the Poodle is between 12 to 15 years.

Despite the long lifespan, the Poodle is a breed that has many health problems. It is important to do your research on this breed to ensure that you are purchasing from a line that is free of inherent diseases.

In addition, the breed does have a skittishness, so it is important to look for stable lines. Look for parents that are not timid or fearful and you should see the same traits in your puppy.

Health problems to be aware of with the Poodle are:

- Addison's Disease
- Allergies
- Bloat, also known as Gastric Dilatation-Volvulus
- Cataracts
- Cushing's Disease, also known as Hyperadrenocorticism
- Diabetes
- Ear Infections
- Epilepsy
- Heart Disease
- Hip Dysplasia
- Hypothyroidism
- Immune Mediated Hemolytic Anemia
- Legg-Perthes Disease
- Optic Nerve Hypoplasia
- Patellar Luxation
- Premature Greying
- Progressive Retinal Atrophy

- Sebaceous Adenitis
- Slipped Stifle
- Van Willebrand's Disease

f) Pros and Cons of the Breed

As you can imagine, there are a number of pros and cons to owning a Poodle, and it is important to weigh them before you bring one home.

Pros of the Poodle are:

- They are usually easy to train as long as you keep training fun.

- They are usually easy to housetrain.

- The breed is quite beautiful and comes in a variety of colors.

- The short coat, with tight curls, is excellent for people with allergies.

- The coat is low-shedding.

- They come in a range of sizes to fit into every enthusiast's needs.

- They are versatile and can live in any dwelling.

- They are very intelligent.

- They have a natural elegance to their movement and are very athletic dogs.

- They are empathetic dogs that are finely tuned to their owner's needs and emotions.

- They are usually polite, playful, and affectionate.

Cons of the Poodle are:

- The coat can be difficult to care for.

- The smaller Poodles often suffer from Small Dog Syndrome.

- The breed is known to be barkers, especially the smaller varieties.

- They can be extremely shy and timid, which can lead to fear and aggression.

- The breed is known to have serious health issues.

- The breed can be overly exuberant and is known for jumping.

- They can become bored easily, which can affect training.

- They require a lot of exercise each day.

In the end, the Poodle is an active breed that can fit into most homes, as long as the owner is prepared for the energy of the breed.

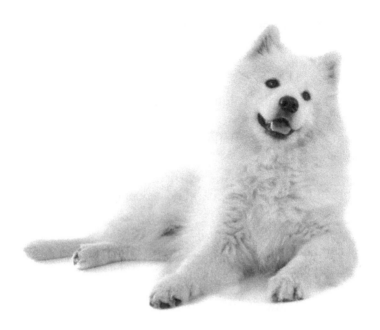

2. The Playful Samoyed

One of the most expensive breeds in the world, the playful Samoyed is quickly charming pet owners and enthusiasts alike. Known for their wonderful temperament, the breed, despite having a longer coat, is known as a hypoallergenic breed.

They are also a strikingly beautiful animal with their white coat and contrasting black nose. But while they are beautiful, the Samoyed is admired more for their loving nature and abundance of energy.

a) History of the Breed

The Samoyed is a working dog that was originally developed to work in a variety of roles. It is unclear when the breed originated; however, we do know that the Samoyed was developed by the Samoyede people. These people were found in Siberia.

Traditionally used as sled dogs, the Samoyed were also used as hunting dogs and herding dogs where they would herd reindeer. The breed also served as bed warmers, and it is this close relationship that has developed the loving temperament of the breed.

By the late 1800s, the Samoyed was discovered by the rest of the world, and they were imported out of Siberia into the early 20th century. The breed was a popular choice for those looking for sled dogs, and they even have the distinction of having traveled with Sir Ernest Shackleton during his expedition to Antarctica.

While they were a very popular breed for adventurers, the breed only had a small following in England and America. It was not until 1909 that the breed standard was created in England and 1924 that it was established in North America.

Today, while the breed can be hard working, the majority of Samoyeds are pampered and beautiful pets.

b) Temperament of the Breed

If you are looking for an intelligent and gentle breed, then you should look no further than the Samoyed. Known for being a happy and friendly breed, the Samoyed is a wonderful family dog that does well with children.

It is a breed that likes to be with their owners, and they are fiercely loyal. They are known for being active dogs, and they do need plenty of exercise. In addition, the breed does need some mental stimulation or they will become bored.

Overall, the Samoyed is an alert breed. They are known as barkers and will often alert their owners to anything they view as suspicious. However, their friendly nature does not make them the ideal guard dog.

Finally, it is important to remember that this is a breed that can run. Many Samoyed have a high prey drive and will often chase things. For that reason, it is important to always have your Samoyed leashed when it is not in a secure yard.

c) Appearance of the Breed

The strikingly rich contrast of black and white coloring is something that many people notice about the breed right away. However, this is a sturdy dog that displays as much athleticism as it does beauty.

With its Spitz-like looks, the Samoyed should have a body that is square in proportion with the height being equal to the length. The body should be muscular, and overall, it should be a compact dog. The tail of the Samoyed should be long but should curl over the back of the dog.

The head of the Samoyed should be wedge-shaped with a tapered muzzle. It should have a definite stop between the forehead and muzzle, and the teeth should be a scissor bite. The eyes should be wide apart and should be almond-shaped.

Overall, you should see a solid dog that is athletic and filled with stamina.

i. Coat

The Samoyed is known for its coat, and it has a very thick double coat. The dog should have a soft undercoat that is very thick. The topcoat should be long and should have a course texture to it. It should stand out from the body, and there should be a thick ruff around the neck. The ruff is more apparent in males than females.

Samoyeds should have a white coat; however, the white can vary in shades and include cream, biscuit, yellow, white with silver tips, and pure white. The eye rims, nose, and lips should be black to provide that startling contrast.

ii. Size

Samoyeds are a medium-sized dog. Males should be slightly larger than females.

Height:
>   Males: 21 to 23.5 inches (53.3 to 59.7 cm)
>   Females: 19 to 21 inches (48.3 to 53.3cm)

Weight:
>   Males: 45 to 60 pounds (20.4 to 27.2kg)
>   Females: 35 to 50 pounds (15.9 to 22.7kg)

d) The Needs of the Breed

Samoyeds, like all breeds, have specific needs that should be taken care of on a daily basis. This includes grooming, exercise, and training. Before you purchase a Samoyed, make sure you understand the needs of the breed.

i. Exercise

The Samoyed is an active breed, so be prepared to give your dog plenty of exercise if you own one. In general, the breed needs about one hour a day of exercise.

In addition, the breed does become bored quickly, so make sure that you give them plenty of intellectual stimulation as well.

This is a breed that does well as a jogging companion; however, their thick coat means they can overheat quickly, so make sure you only exercise them during cooler times of the day.

ii. Living Conditions

When it comes to living conditions, the Samoyed does best in a home with a small yard so they can expel their energy. That being said, the Samoyed can do okay in an apartment, but they will need plenty of exercise, as they tend to be very active indoors.

iii. Ease of Training

Training can be a wonderful experience with the Samoyed. They are very intelligent and will learn quickly with the right setting. However, they can become bored with repetitive training and may become a challenge in that case.

The best type of training to use with the Samoyed is positive reinforcement since they are happy to work for their people. Remember to socialize this breed as they can become aloof with strangers. They are not usually a good match for homes with small pets as they can have a high prey drive if they are not raised with smaller pets.

iv. Grooming Requirements

Grooming the Samoyed is not for the faint of heart. This breed has a very thick coat that needs to be brushed daily to keep the hair down. And you should expect a lot of hair. While the breed is considered to be hypoallergenic since it produces a small amount of the allergen, it does shed heavily, especially in warmer climates.

Bathing should be done weekly to keep the coat bright. In addition to bathing and brushing, you will need to clean the ears weekly. The nails will also need to be trimmed at least once per month, and you should trim the hair around footpads and ears if it is growing too much.

e) Health of the Breed

The average lifespan of the Samoyed is between 12 to 15 years.

It is a fairly hardy breed; however, they have a high incidence of hip dysplasia, which can greatly affect the dog's quality and length of life. It is important to do your research on this breed to ensure that you are purchasing from a line that is free of inherent diseases.

Health problems to be aware of with the Samoyed are:

- Cancer
- Diabetes Mellitus
- Glaucoma
- Hip Dysplasia
- Hypothyroidism
- Progressive Retinal Atrophy
- Samoyed Hereditary Ghlomerulopathy
- Subvalvular Aortic Stenosis

f) Pros and Cons of the Breed

As you can imagine, there are a number of pros and cons to owning a Samoyed, and it is important to weigh them before you bring one home.

Pros of the Samoyed are:

- They are strikingly beautiful dogs that have a fox-like appearance.

- They are loving companions that do well in a family setting.

- The Samoyed is excellent with children.

- Their energy makes them a perfect pet for a busy owner who enjoys walks and jogging.

- They will get along with everyone.

- The Samoyed is an alert dog, and they make excellent watchdogs, as they will alert you to something suspicious.

- Generally, the Samoyed is easy to train and is very intelligent.

Cons of the Samoyed are:

- This is a breed that requires a lot of grooming.

- The Samoyed is a heavy shedder, especially when it lives in warmer climates.

- They are known for being stubborn and can be difficult to train if they find training boring.

- They are active dogs that need a lot of exercise.

- The Samoyed can be prone to bad habits such as jumping.

- They can become problem barkers.

- The Samoyed thrives when they are with family and may become destructive if left alone too much.

Overall, the Samoyed is a wonderful dog that fits into a family that has an active lifestyle. They do better in homes than apartments, but with proper care, they can live just about anywhere.

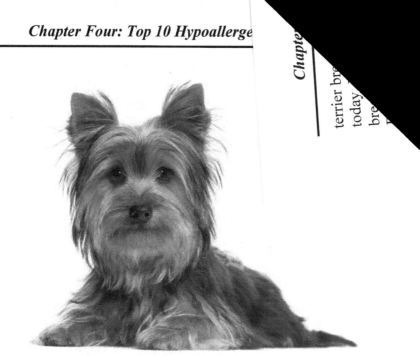

3. The Tiny Yorkshire Terrier

It may be a tiny dog, but the Yorkshire Terrier is a breed that has huge personality. The breed is known for being a brave and energetic breed that gets along well with everyone. They love their owners and will protect them without any regard for their own size or safety.

The breed is a hypoallergenic breed simply because of its size -- the Yorkshire Terrier does not produce a lot of dander, so most allergy sufferers can do very well with the breed.

a) History of the Breed

The Yorkshire Terrier is a breed of terrier that was developed in England. They were believed to have been produced when Scottish workers immigrated to Yorkshire looking for work during the Industrial Revolution.

As they migrated, they brought with them several terrier breeds, and it is believed that these terrier breeds crossed with other eds to produce the Yorkshire Terrier as we know it Breeds that are believed to have been used in creating this ed are the Waterside Terrier, Clydesdale Terrier, English Black and Tan Toy Terrier, and the Skye Terrier. The result was a small dog that became known as the Broken Haired Scotch Terrier.

By 1861, the breed was established, but it wasn't until Huddersfield Ben, a small Broken Haired Scotch Terrier, became a popular site on the show dog circuit. The dog became one of the more popular stud dogs, and many Yorkshire Terriers can be traced back to Huddersfield Ben.

In 1870, the name of the breed was switched to Yorkshire Terrier, and by 1874, the breed was accepted by the British Kennel Club. In North America, the Yorkshire Terrier was accepted by the AKC in 1878.

b) Temperament of the Breed

Adventurous, brave, and energetic, the Yorkshire Terrier is almost oblivious to its diminutive size. They are always ready for the next adventure, and this can often keep their owners busy.

The breed is usually very affectionate, and they thrive when they are with their family. They are usually an intelligent breed that is quite clever at times.

Fiercely loyal, they can become overprotective if they feel they need to. They are not afraid of any other dog or threat, despite their size, and they can be quite bossy.

The breed can do well with children since they are so affectionate; however, they are not recommended for homes with young children since they can be easily injured.

c) Appearance of the Breed

The Yorkshire Terrier is a toy-sized breed of dog and should be very small. They should be delicate but should still have a robust structure to them. The body should be slightly longer than tall, and the tail should be medium in length. It is important to note that the tail is often docked; however, in some areas in Europe, it is illegal, so the Yorkshire Terrier will have a full tail in those areas.

The head should be flat on the top while the muzzle should be medium in width. The muzzle should not taper. The ears should be held erect and should be v-shaped.

i. Coat

Silky, long, and beautiful are often words used to describe the coat of the Yorkshire Terrier, and they are all correct. The coat should be a single coat, and it should be straight.

Many owners keep the coat clipped short; however, if it is allowed to grow to full length, it should reach the floor. The coat should be silky to the touch, and there should be an abundance of hair on the head.

One interesting note about the Yorkshire Terrier is that all puppies are born with a black coat. As the puppy gets older, the coat begins to change color to take on the tan coat with steel blue on the tail and back.

ii. Size

The Yorkshire Terrier is a very small dog and has the distinction of being one of the smallest breeds of dogs. In fact, several Yorkshire Terriers broke world records regarding size. Males and females tend to be about the same size.

Height:

6 to 7 inches (15.2 to 17.8cm)

Weight:

4 to 7 pounds (1.8 to 3.2kg)

d) The Needs of the Breed

Although they have a small size, the Yorkshire Terrier does have many daily needs that new owners should be aware of. This includes grooming, exercise, and training.

i. Exercise

Despite being a toy breed, the Yorkshire Terrier has a lot of energy and will need about 30 minutes of exercise a day. In addition, they love playing games and will spend a lot of time chasing balls through the house if you let them.

One word of caution with the Yorkshire Terrier is that it is a terrier breed, and they do have a high prey drive. They will chase animals they feel is prey, so keep them leashed when they are not in a secure area.

Finally, remember that their small size makes them ideal for predators to attack, so never leave them unattended outside.

ii. Living Conditions

Because of their size, the Yorkshire Terrier can live in any dwelling. They do well in apartments, but they can be problem barkers, so make sure your building does not have noise restrictions.

iii. Ease of Training

The Yorkshire Terrier can be an easy dog to train; however, they do have the terrier tenacity, so you may have some problems with training if you are not consistent.

One of the biggest problems with Yorkshire Terriers is that they are often babied. This leads to problems such as Small Dog Syndrome. When this occurs, you may have to deal with destructive behavior, problem barking, and a host of other problems. To avoid this, treat your Yorkshire Terrier like a dog and give it clear rules. Trust me; despite their size, they can quickly rule the house if they are allowed to.

iv. Grooming Requirements

Grooming varies depending on how you keep your dog's coat. If you choose a puppy trim, you will need to have the dog's coat shaved every 4 to 6 weeks. In addition, you will need to brush the dog's coat every day or every other day. This will keep it from matting.

If you keep your dog in its full coat, you will need to brush the coat daily. In addition, the hair on the head will need to either be trimmed to keep it out of the dog's eyes or held up with an elastic band.

The coat should be washed weekly to keep it in top condition. In addition, when you are bathing your dog, make sure that you use a conditioner on the coat. This will help keep it tangle-free.

Finally, as with all dogs, you will need to clean the ears weekly. The nails will also need to be trimmed at least once per month. Make sure you brush the Yorkshire Terrier's teeth, as they are prone to tooth issues.

e) Health of the Breed

The average lifespan of the Yorkshire Terrier is between 12 to 15 years.

This toy-sized breed is a healthy one; however, their popularity has seen a rise in some serious health problems. It is important to do your research on this breed to ensure that you are purchasing from a line that is free of inherent diseases.

Health problems to be aware of with the Yorkshire Terrier are:

- Collapsed Trachea
- Eye Infections
- Gum Infections
- Hypoglycemia
- Patellar Luxation
- Progressive Retinal Atrophy
- Portosystemic Shunt
- Reverse Sneezing

f) Pros and Cons of the Breed

As you can imagine, there are a number of pros and cons to owning a Yorkshire Terrier, and it is important to weigh them before you bring one home.

Pros of the Yorkshire Terrier are:

- They are small dogs that can live anywhere.

- They are very low shedders, so they do not produce a lot of hair.

- Their small size makes them ideal for allergy sufferers.

- They are active dogs, but they don't need a lot of exercise.

- They are usually very inquisitive and can be a joy to own.

- They are brave dogs that are fiercely loyal.

- They are excellent watchdogs as they will alert bark.

Cons of the Yorkshire Terrier are:

- They can develop Small Dog Syndrome, which can lead to many behavior problems.

- They need to be properly socialized or they can become high strung.

- They are difficult to housetrain.

- They are very delicate and can be easily injured.

- They have a high prey drive and will run after something without too much thought to their own safety.

- The breed needs to be groomed a lot, and their coat can be difficult to care for.

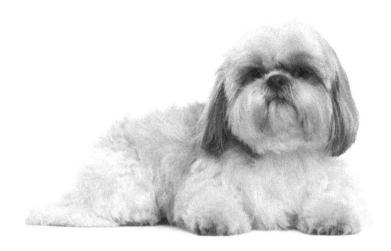

4. The Friendly Shih Tzu

Pronounced SHē 'dzoo, the Shih Tzu is a breed that has a lot of admirers -- not only for its beauty but also for its temperament. The breed is known for being a friendly and affectionate companion.

They are a versatile breed that does well in a range of dwellings and are always happy to be with their owners.

a) History of the Breed

The Shih Tzu is a breed that is believed to be one of the oldest breeds alive today. In fact, it is believed that the breed may have been developed before the 600 ADs, and there are paintings of that time that show similar-looking dogs.

The breed is believed to have been the result of crossing the Lhasa Apso with the Pekingese, although it is unclear of whether this was done in Tibet or in China. What we do know is that the Shih Tzu became a very popular breed with Chinese royalty.

Between the 1700s and 1800s, it is believed that the breed fell out of favor; however, when the Empress Tzu Hsi ruled China, she fell in love with the breed. It is her interest in the breed that saw its resurgence during the late 1800s.

The first Shih Tzus to be imported from China was in 1928, and the breed quickly became a favorite to many. The breed was recognized by the AKC in 1969.

b) Temperament of the Breed

Affectionate, lively, and happy, there is a lot of personality packed into such a small package. The Shih Tzu is a friendly little dog that is usually very gentle. They are known for being an excellent breed for families; however, they are better suited for homes with older children due to their size.

The breed is usually very loyal to their family, and while they will alert bark, they are friendly with strangers. The breed is intelligent, and they have a spunky nature that can get them into trouble now and then.

c) Appearance of the Breed

The Shih Tzu is a small breed of dog that should have a rectangular body that is slightly longer than it is tall. Overall, while it is a toy-sized breed, it should have the appearance and structure of a sturdy dog. The back should be level, and the tail should be carried over the back.

The head of the Shih Tzu should be broad and should have a round shape. The muzzle should be very short and should have a well defined stop.

i. Coat

A long, double coat covers the Shih Tzu, and it should be very thick. The hair should consist of a short, soft undercoat and a long top coat. The top coat should be abundant and should flow down the body of the dog. It should have enough hair on the top of the head to create a topknot, and there should be a mustache and beard on the face.

Shih Tzus come in a range of colors, including red and white, black, grey and white, and black and white; however, you can find them in any color.

ii. Size

The Shih Tzu is a toy-sized breed of dog with males and females being roughly the same size.

Height:
>   9 to 10 inches (22.7 to 25.4cm)

Weight:
>   9 to 16 pounds (4.1 to 7.3kg)

d) The Needs of the Breed

Shih Tzus, like all breeds, have specific needs that should be taken care of on a daily basis. This includes grooming, exercise, and training. Before you purchase a Shih Tzu, make sure you understand the needs of the breed.

i. Exercise

The Shih Tzu doesn't require a lot of exercise, and many can meet their exercise needs simply by playing a game of fetch in the home. That being said, the breed does enjoy going for walks and should have at least 30 minutes of exercise every day.

ii. Living Conditions

The breed is an excellent choice for people who live in apartments. They can be prone to barking, so make sure you check your building's noise restrictions if you own one.

iii. Ease of Training

Easy to train, the Shih Tzu is usually eager to please and will take to training quickly. Owners should avoid babying the breed as they can suffer from Small Dog Syndrome. When this occurs, you may have to deal with destructive behavior, problem barking, and a host of other problems.

To avoid Small Dog Syndrome, place firm and consistent rules in the house. Socialization should be done with the Shih Tzu, but they usually get along well with everyone.

iv. Grooming Requirements

Grooming requirements can vary depending on how you keep the dog's coat. If you keep it clipped in a puppy cut, grooming is quite easy and simply requires brushing every few days. Bathing with the cut coat can be left to when the dog is clipped, which is every 4 to 6 weeks.

If you are keeping the Shih Tzu in a full coat, grooming becomes more of a challenge. The coat should be brushed on a daily basis, and it will need to be bathed about once per week. In addition, you will either have to trim the hair on the forehead or create a topknot daily so the hair is not in the dog's eyes.

Another important aspect of the Shih Tzu grooming, regardless of coat, is eye care. Eyes should be wiped clean on a daily basis and it may be important to add drops to the eye, but only if your vet recommends it. Shih Tzus have many eye problems.

Finally, teeth should be brushed weekly, and nails should be trimmed on a monthly basis. Ears should be cleaned every week.

e) Health of the Breed

The average lifespan of the Shih Tzu is between 14 to 15 years.

While many lines are healthy, the breed has several serious health conditions. It is important to do your research on this breed to ensure that you are purchasing from a line that is free of inherent diseases.

Health problems to be aware of with the Shih Tzu are:

- Allergies
- Bladder Infections
- Bladder Stones
- Distichiasis
- Ear Infections
- Ectopia Cilia
- Gum Disease
- Hip Dysplasia
- Juvenile Renal Dysplasia
- Keratitis
- Keratoconjunctivitis Sicca
- Patellar Luxation
- Portosystemic Liver Shunt
- Progressive Retinal Atrophy
- Proptosis
- Retained Baby Teeth
- Reverse Sneezing
- Snuffles
- Umbilical Hernia

f) Pros and Cons of the Breed

As you can imagine, there are a number of pros and cons to owning a Shih Tzu, and it is important to weigh them before you bring one home.

Pros of the Shih Tzu are:

- While the breed barks, it is considered to be a quieter small breed.

- They are very friendly dogs that get along well with others.

- They are good with children.

- The breed is a low shedder, so it is an excellent breed for people with allergies.

- The Shih Tzu only requires moderate exercise.

- They can live in any setting and make excellent apartment pets.

- Their sturdy bodies make them less delicate small dogs.

Cons of the Shih Tzu are:

- Training can be a challenge as the Shih Tzu is known for being stubborn.

- The coat can be difficult to care for, and they require daily grooming.

- They can have difficulties housetraining.

- The breed can suffer from Small Dog Syndrome, which can lead to may behavior problems.

- They can have a lot of health problems.

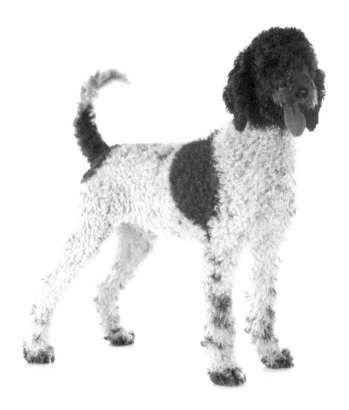

5. The Clown Like Portuguese Water Dog

Funny, and silly, the Portuguese Water Dog is a breed that often claims the hearts of anyone who meets them.

This is a breed that loves being with people, and they are exceptional family pets. In addition, the low-shedding coat makes them perfect for allergy sufferers.

a) History of the Breed

Native to Portugal, the Portuguese Water Dog is a breed that was developed to work alongside fishermen. Originally, the breed was used to retrieve gear from the water and take messages from the boat; however, today, the breed is utilized in many ways, including as a family pet.

The breed is believed to have been developed from the same breed that created the Poodle. It is unclear when the breed was developed; however, we do know that in the 1930s, the breed began to decline due to not being used for their original purpose.

However, in the late 1960s, more interest went into saving the breed, and the Portuguese Water Dog began to flourish again. In 1972, the Portuguese Water Dog Club of America was founded, and by 1983, they were accepted by the AKC. Today, the breed has a large following and ranks in the top 50 dog breeds according to the AKC.

b) Temperament of the Breed

Known for their clown-like nature, the Portuguese Water Dog is an amusing breed that is wonderful with children. The breed is often a very gentle breed that loves to play.

Their jovial temperament often leaves their owners laughing, and they love being with their family. They are an extremely loyal breed that is known as being very intelligent. In fact, sometimes their intelligence can make them a bit hard to handle, especially during training, but if they are having fun, then they are easy to train.

The breed loves water, and while they can be very calm, they need plenty of exercise.

c) Appearance of the Breed

The Portuguese Water Dog is a beautiful dog that should have a sturdy appearance. They are usually muscular and built for working, especially swimming. The body should be slightly rectangular, with the body longer than the dog is tall. The back should be level, and the tail should taper and be carried high.

The head of the Portuguese Water Dog should be broad with a slightly long muzzle. The ears should be set high on the head and should be hanging and heart-shaped.

i. Coat

The Portuguese Water Dog should have a single-layered coat that is very thick. The texture should range between curly to wavy.

The color of the coat can be black, brown, or white. Parti color is a popular color combination and is two colors. These are white with black spots, black with white markings, or brown with white markings. In the black and brown coat, the markings can also be silver or grey.

ii. Size

The Portuguese Water Dog is a medium-sized breed of dog.

Height:
Males: 20 to 22 inches (50.8 to 55.9 cm)
Females: 17 to 20 inches (43.2 to 50.8cm)

Weight:
Males: 42 to 55 pounds (19.1 to 25kg)
Females: 35 to 49 pounds (15.9 to 22.2kg)

d) The Needs of the Breed

Portuguese Water Dogs, like all breeds, have specific needs that should be taken care of on a daily basis. This includes grooming, exercise, and training. Before you purchase a Portuguese Water Dog, make sure you understand the needs of the breed.

i. Exercise

The Portuguese Water Dog is an active breed that does require a lot of exercise. Expect to give them at least an hour of exercise each day. The breed does make excellent jogging companions because of their energy levels.

In addition to daily walks, make sure you give your Portuguese Water Dog time to swim, run off leash, and problem solve. Without proper exercise, a Portuguese Water Dog can become destructive.

ii. Living Conditions

The ideal living condition for a Portuguese Water Dog is in a home with a fenced yard so they can expel their energy. However, if you properly exercise the breed, they can do okay in apartments, but exercise is a must.

iii. Ease of Training

Portuguese Water Dogs can be very easy to train as the breed is eager to please. However, it is important to remember that the breed is playful and loves to clown around, so make sure you are patient with them.

While they are usually very friendly dogs, socialization is important so they do not become fearful or aggressive.

iv. Grooming Requirements

When it comes to grooming, the Portuguese Water Dog is generally very easy to care for. The coat is a slow growing coat, and it is customary to clip the dog's coat so it is only an inch long.

There are actually two different cuts that you can get for the Portuguese Water Dog. One is where the face and back end of the dog is shaved and the rest of the coat is clipped. The other is where the entire dog is clipped to about an inch in length. Most pet owners choose the latter clip.

Clipping should be done every 6 to 8 weeks. Bathing only needs to be done about once a month. Ears should be cleaned weekly, and teeth should be brushed weekly as well. Nails should be clipped monthly.

e) Health of the Breed

The average lifespan of the Portuguese Water Dog is between 10 to 14 years.

The breed is considered to be very healthy; however, with the increase in popularity, some diseases have begun to appear in the breed. It is important to do your research on this breed to ensure that you are purchasing from a line that is free of inherent diseases.

Health problems to be aware of with the Portuguese Water Dog are:

- Hip Dysplasia
- Juvenile Dilated Cardiomyopathy
- Progressive Retinal Atrophy
- Storage Disease

f) Pros and Cons of the Breed

As you can imagine, there are a number of pros and cons to owning a Portuguese Water Dog, and it is important to weigh them before you bring one home.

Pros of the Portuguese Water Dog are:

- They are an affectionate breed that is friendly with everyone.

- They do very well with children and in homes with an active family.

- The Portuguese Water Dog is an active dog that can make an excellent jogging companion.

- They have a coat that doesn't require a lot of maintenance.

- The breed is an excellent watchdog as they will alert bark.

- They are good with other pets in the home.

- The breed is considered to be a low- to non-shedding breed.

- They are quite comical and known for being clown-like.

Cons of the Portuguese Water Dog are:

- This is a breed with a lot of energy, so expect a lot of exercise.

- They are prone to bad behaviors such as jumping and being overly rowdy.

- They can be difficult to train if they are bored, and they really need a strong owner.

- The Portuguese Water Dog can be destructive when it is not properly exercised or stimulated.

- The breed can be quite mouthy, which means they are prone to destructive chewing and nipping.

- They do better in homes where there is a yard to play in. It is not the best breed for apartments.

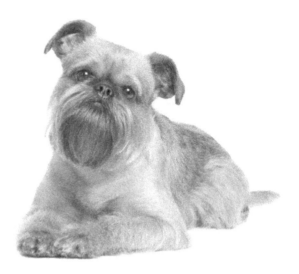

6. The Fearless Brussels Griffon

With the tenacity often seen in Terrier breeds, the Brussels Griffon is a friendly, cheerful, and fearless breed. It is a toy-sized breed, but what they lack in size, they definitely make up for in personality.

The breed is an amazing choice for allergy sufferers because the two coat varieties you find in this breed shed very little. In addition, their small size means that less allergens are produced by the dog.

a) History of the Breed

Originally developed in Belgium, the Brussels Griffon did not start out as a companion. Instead, the breed was developed to kill vermin in stables. The breed is believed to have been developed by crossing the English Toy Spaniel, the Affenpinscher, and the Pug.

While it was originally a working dog, the breed quickly captured the hearts of many and became a popular companion breed. The first breed standard was developed in 1883 for the Brussels Griffon, and the breed was imported into England in the 1890s. In addition, the breed quickly made its way to North America and was accepted by the AKC in 1900.

Today, the breed has become a popular family pet and continues to entertain many owners.

b) Temperament of the Breed

An intelligent breed, the Brussels Griffon is a bright-eyed dog that is full of personality. Known as being cheerful, the breed is a wonderful companion breed. They are very affectionate with their owners, and overall, the Brussels Griffon gets along well with everyone.

They are little spitfires as well. The breed can be bossy if they are allowed to be; however, when they are given clear rules, the Brussels Griffon is a wonderful breed that is happy sitting with their owners or performing tricks for them.

c) Appearance of the Breed

The Brussels Griffon is a funny little dog when it comes to appearance. It is a toy-sized breed of dog that has a robust look to it. The breed should be slightly rectangular in shape and should have medium length legs. The head should be domed with a very short muzzle. Eyes should be wide, and the ears should be set high. In some countries, the ears will be cropped to stand erect, but the natural ears are semi-erect.

i. Coat

The Brussels Griffon can be found in two different coat types. The first coat type is the smooth coat. In this variety, the coat should be very short and straight. It should have a coarse texture to it and should be tight to the skin. It should be glossy.

The second coat type is the rough coat. This should be a coat with a dense, wiry texture. The coat should be longer than the short, and there should be a full beard, mustache, and bushy eyebrows.

Brussels Griffons can be found in several colors, including solid black, solid red, black and tan, and belge, which is a mixture of red-brown and black.

ii. Size

Brussels Griffons are a toy-sized breed of dog with males and females being roughly the same size.

Height:
> 7 to 8 inches (17.8 to 20.3cm)

Weight:
> 6 to 12 pounds (2.72 to 5.4kg)

d) The Needs of the Breed

Brussels Griffons, like all breeds, have specific needs that should be taken care of on a daily basis. This includes grooming, exercise, and training. Before you purchase a Brussels Griffon, make sure you understand the needs of the breed.

i. Exercise

Although it is a toy-sized breed, the Brussels Griffon does have a fair amount of energy. For that reason, they will need to be exercised daily, usually for about a half hour a day.

When they are not in a secure area, keep the Brussels Griffon on leash as they can be easily injured if they run away. The breed should always be monitored, even when they are in a fenced yard as their small size puts them at risk for predator attacks.

ii. Living Conditions

The Brussels Griffon is a very versatile breed that can live just about anywhere. They do very well in apartments. That being said, they are not recommended for homes with small children because of their size.

iii. Ease of Training

The Brussels Griffon is an intelligent breed that is usually very easy to train. They do very well with positive reinforcement and will learn quickly.

Owners should avoid babying the breed as they can suffer from Small Dog Syndrome. When this occurs, you may have to deal with destructive behavior, problem barking, and a host of other problems.

To avoid Small Dog Syndrome, place firm and consistent rules in the house.

iv. Grooming Requirements

Grooming requirements differ depending on the coat type of your Brussels Griffon. In general, the smooth coated Brussels Griffon is very easy to groom. A wipe down with a damp cloth is usually all that is needed to keep the dog looking its best.

The rough coated Brussels Griffon is harder. The coats should be brushed weekly to keep it free of tangles. In addition, the coat should be hand stripped every few months. This is done by gently pulling out loose hairs with a stripping comb.

Bathing should be done as needed, usually about once per month. Eyes should be washed weekly, and the ears should be as well. Nails should be clipped monthly.

e) Health of the Breed

The average lifespan of the Brussels Griffon is between 12 to 15 years.

The breed is considered to be a healthy breed, but they do have some serious health problems potential owners should be aware of. It is important to do your research on this breed to ensure that you are purchasing from a line that is free of inherent diseases.

Health problems to be aware of with the Brussels Griffon are:

- Allergies
- Eye Infections
- Hip Dysplasia
- Patellar Luxation

f) Pros and Cons of the Breed

As you can imagine, there are a number of pros and cons to owning a Brussels Griffon, and it is important to weigh them before you bring one home.

Pros of the Brussels Griffon are:

- They are a breed that can live just about anywhere.

- The breed is known for being a low-shedding breed, although the shorter coat sheds more than the longer coat.

- The breed is quite spunky and can be fearless.

- They are a serious, but the seriousness is quite endearing.

- They can do well with older children; however, their small size makes them unsuitable for younger children.

- They don't require a lot of exercise.

- The wiry coat can be easy to care for.

Cons of the Brussels Griffon are:

- The breed can be quite fragile since they are so small.

- There is a high demand for Brussels Griffon, so there can be a long wait to own one.

- They can suffer from Small Dog Syndrome, which can lead to destructive behaviors.

- The breed can be a problem barker.

- They can be difficult to housetrain.

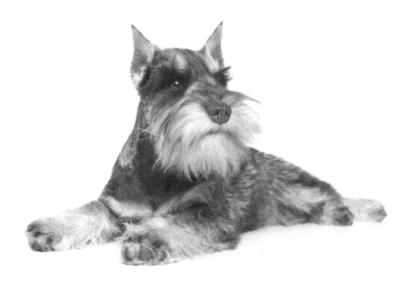

7. The Vigilant Schnauzer

Serious, intelligent, and charming, the Schnauzer is a popular breed for allergy sufferers.

The low-shedding coat is one of the many traits that people find appealing. One of the most, however, is that there are three varieties, so whether you are looking for a little dog or a large one, there is a Schnauzer to fit your needs.

a) History of the Breed

The history of the Schnauzer differs slightly depending on the actual variety that you are looking at. The first Schnauzer breed is believed to be the Standard Schnauzer.

This breed can be traced back to the early 1500s and were developed in Germany. They were used as guard dogs for livestock and homesteads and were also successful vermin hunters.

Breeding for the Schnauzer became standardized in the mid-1800s, and the breed became quite popular. During WWII, the breed was commonly used as a messenger dog and in Germany for police work.

The Standard Schnauzer was accepted into the AKC in 1945.

The Giant Schnauzer was also developed in Germany and was the result of crossing the Standard Schnauzer with the Great Dane and possibly the Bouvier des Flandres. The breed was developed to drive cattle and to also be a guard dog. The breed was originally known as the munchener but eventually given the name of Giant Schnauzer.

While the breed is still fairly uncommon, it was accepted by the AKC in 1930, and while it was used as a driving dog, the working nature of the Giant Schnauzer has made it an excellent police dog.

The Miniature Schnauzer was also developed by crossing the Standard Schnauzer with the Affenpinscher and Miniature Pinscher. It is also believed that the Poodle and the Pomeranian was also introduced in the lines.

The breed was originally used as ratters and it was only in 1888 that the first documented Miniature Schnauzer was seen. The breed came close to extinction during WWII; however, after the war, the popularity of the breed grew.

The breed was first accepted by the AKC in 1926, and today, it is ranked in the top 20 of most popular dog breeds.

b) Temperament of the Breed

The Schnauzer is an intelligent breed that is known for being a serious but loving companion.

The breed is slightly different depending on the size. Giant Schnauzers take the role of protector very seriously. They will risk their life for their family, and while they are very loving, they are also hard-working.

The Standard Schnauzer is very similar in temperament; however, they are often described as being a stubborn breed. They are usually very territorial and make excellent watchdogs. The breed is also very inquisitive, and this can lead them to trouble.

Finally, the Miniature Schnauzer is the breed that is a little more carefree than the other two varieties of Schnauzer. They have a terrier temperament and are quite adventurous and courageous. The breed loves to be in the middle of the family and thrives when they are with those they love.

c) Appearance of the Breed

The Schnauzer has three varieties that range from small to large. All of the variations should be robust dogs that have a square body that is the same length as height. The overall back should be level, and it should have a look of a working dog.

The head should be rectangular in shape with a muzzle that is the same length as the head. The eyes of the Schnauzer should show its intelligence and should be medium-sized. The ears should be carried high on the head and should be v-shaped when they are not cropped.

i. Coat

The Schnauzer should have a thick double coat. This should consist of a soft, dense undercoat and a wiry top coat. The top coat should be longer than the undercoat, but it is usually clipped short. All of the Schnauzer varieties should have a bushy beard and mustache as well as bushy eyebrows.

The coat colors for Giant Schnauzer and Standard Schnauzer can either be black or salt and pepper. The Miniature Schnauzer can be black, salt and pepper, white, or black and silver.

ii. Size

There are three different sizes for the Schnauzer; however, all three sizes have the same structure, temperament, and needs. It should be noted that female Schnauzers tend to be smaller than males.

The sizes are:

Miniature:
> 12 to 14 inches (30.48 to 35.6cm) in height
> 10 to 15 pounds (4.5 to 6.8kg) in weight

Standard:
> 17 to 20 inches (43.2 to 50.8cm) in height
> 30 to 45 pounds (13.6 to 20.4kg) in weight

Giant:
> 26 to 28 inches (66.0 to 71.1cm) or more in height
> 55 to 105 pounds (24.9 to 47.6kg) in weight

d) The Needs of the Breed

Schnauzers, like all breeds, have specific needs that should be taken care of on a daily basis. This includes grooming, exercise, and training. Before you purchase a Schnauzer, make sure you understand the needs of the breed.

i. Exercise

Regardless of size, the Schnauzer is an energetic breed that does require ample exercise. They should have at least an hour of exercise per day. In addition, this breed is an intelligent breed so make sure you give them puzzle toys to keep them entertained. A bored and under-exercised Schnauzer can be quite destructive.

ii. Living Conditions

The Miniature Schnauzer and Standard Schnauzer does very well in apartments and can live in any type of dwelling. However, the Giant Schnauzer is not suitable for apartments as they need a yard to run in.

Schnauzers, in general, are not always that accepting of children, so they do much better in homes with no children or older children.

iii. Ease of Training

Since the Schnauzer is an intelligent breed, they can be an easier breed to train. That being said, the Miniature and Standard Schnauzers are usually eager to please and will learn quickly.

The Giant Schnauzer, however, is a more difficult breed to train. While they are intelligent, they can be stubborn and often do things when they choose to. They need an owner who is firm and consistent.

All Schnauzers need ample socialization as they can be very suspicious of strangers. They make excellent watchdogs, and the Giant Schnauzer makes an excellent guard dog. If they are not properly socialized, they can become aggressive toward people and other animals.

iv. Grooming Requirements

The Schnauzer is generally an easy breed to groom. Brushing should be done several times a week to keep the coat in top condition.

Generally, the coat is clipped all over the dog several times a year to keep it about an inch to a half inch in length. This makes the coat more manageable. If you are keeping the dog in show coat, you would keep the hair longer on the under body and short on the top of the body.

Like the Brussels Griffon, you can also hand strip the coat, which is pulling out loose hairs with a stripping comb, several times per year.

Bathing only needs to be done when the dog needs it, usually about once per month. Ears should be cleaned weekly, and nails should be trimmed once or twice a month.

e) Health of the Breed

The average lifespan of a Schnauzer is between 12 to 15 years. It is important to note that the Standard and Miniature Schnauzer have longer lifespans than the Giant, with many Standard and Miniature Schnauzers living over 15 years.

All of the varieties are fairly healthy, but they do have some serious health problems potential owners should be aware of. It is interesting to note that the Standard Schnauzer appears to be the variety that has very few health problems. It is important to do your research on this breed to ensure that you are purchasing from a line that is free of inherent diseases.

Health problems to be aware of with the Schnauzer are:

- Autoimmune Thyroiditis
- Cataracts
- Entropion
- Hip Dysplasia
- Myotonia Congenita
- Osteochondrosis Dissecans
- Progressive Retinal Atrophy
- Squamous Cell Carcinoma
- Urinary Stones
- Von Willebrand's Disease

- Congenital Megaesophagus

f) Pros and Cons of the Breed

As you can imagine, there are a number of pros and cons to owning a Schnauzer, and it is important to weigh them before you bring one home.

Pros of the Schnauzer are:

- The breed can be found in three sizes, which makes it perfect for a range of households.

- They are serious dogs that are loyal to their families.

- They can be trained to do a range of jobs.

- They are hardworking, and the larger breed is an ideal jogging companion since it has ample energy.

- Their wiry coat is generally easy to care for; however, it does need to be regularly maintained.

- They are a light- to non-shedding breed, so they are perfect for allergy sufferers.

- The breed is friendly with their family.

- They are excellent watchdogs and will be quite serious about protecting their family.

Cons of the Schnauzer are:

- High energy can mean that the breed has high exercise needs.

- They can be difficult to train as the Schnauzer has a mind of its own.

- Not for new or inexperienced owners.

- They often prefer adults to children and are not always the ideal breed for homes with young children.

- They can be very aggressive toward other dogs and animals, so socialization is a must.

- They need ample intellectual stimulation as they become bored easily.

- They can be destructive when bored.

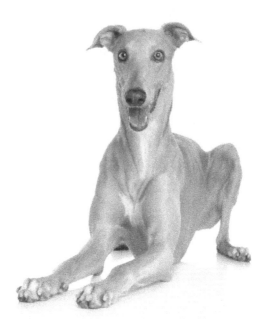

8. The Quick Italian Greyhound

The Italian Greyhound is a small breed of dog that is known for their sighthound appearance that is both elegant and graceful. The breed is a loving companion and is a sensitive soul. They do well in a range of different settings but really thrive in homes that are calm and stable.

a) History of the Breed

When it comes to history, the Italian Greyhound is a breed with a long one. Believed to have been developed millennia ago, depictions of the breed have been found on artifacts that are over 2,000 years old. In fact, there is much evidence to show that the small Greyhound-like dogs have been a prized companion to many.

While the breed can be traced back to Ancient Greece where it was a hunting dog for small rodents, it wasn't until the middle ages when it was established. During that time, the Italian

Greyhound was a popular dog breed for the aristocracy. By the 1600s, the breed was imported to England, where it became a favorite of many royals, including Queen Victoria.

The breed was accepted by the AKC in 1886, but during the World Wars, the breed declined in numbers. However, after the war, the Italian Greyhound grew in popularity and continues to be a popular breed today.

b) Temperament of the Breed

Sensitive and intelligent are two words that are commonly used to describe the Italian Greyhound. This little breed is a very intelligent companion that thrives when they can be with the people they love.

They are usually very affectionate and are a Velcro breed that needs to be by their owner's side. They are usually very polite; however, they can be quite shy with strangers.

The Italian Greyhound is usually a playful companion. It is important to note that the Italian Greyhound can be very sensitive, and harsh corrections or mistreatment can shut the breed down.

c) Appearance of the Breed

The Italian Greyhound is a small-sized breed of dog that looks very similar to the Greyhound. They should be a slender dog with a very narrow appearance. The body should be slightly longer than they are tall, and they should be lean. The body should be fine-boned, but they should still appear athletic and graceful with a long neck.

A wedged-shape head should taper to a point on the muzzle. The eyes should be large and alert. The small ears should be held angled slightly but should be erect. The tail of the Italian Greyhound should be long and tapered to a point.

i. Coat

The Italian Greyhound has a single coat that is very short and lies close to the body. The coat should be glossy and never dull.

Coat colors can vary, and the breed can be found in all colors. The most common are red, black, cream, blue, fawn, grey, or slate grey. They can be solid; however, white markings on the chest and feet are commonly seen. While it is not an accepted coloration in the breed standard, you can find brindle as well as black and tan colored Italian Greyhounds.

ii. Size

Italian Greyhounds are a small breed of dog. They fall into a small weight category; however, it should be noted that the breed is split into two groups: dogs that are under 8 pounds (3.6kg) and dogs that are over 8 pounds (3.6kg). Males and females should be roughly the same in height and weight.

Height:
12 to 15 inches (30.5 to 38.1cm)

Weight:
6 to 10 pounds (2.7 to 4.5kg)

d) The Needs of the Breed

Italian Greyhounds, like all breeds, have specific needs that should be taken care of on a daily basis. This includes grooming, exercise, and training. Before you purchase an Italian Greyhound, make sure you understand the needs of the breed.

i. Exercise

Italian Greyhounds are an active breed, and they do need a lot of exercise. On average, your Italian Greyhound should be exercised about an hour a day. They should not be trusted off leash when they are not in a secure area as they do have a high prey drive and will chase things. And these little dogs are extremely fast!

ii. Living Conditions

The Italian Greyhound can do well in any dwelling and are excellent companions for people living in apartments. The do have high energy, so a home with a small fenced yard is an ideal fit for this breed.

iii. Ease of Training

Italian Greyhounds are easy to train as long as you do not use harsh correction on them. Harsh correction will shut the dog down and will make training next to impossible. Instead, use positive reinforcement and keep training fun.

In addition to training, make sure you socialize the Italian Greyhound. They can be very timid around strangers, so they need to be socialized enough to accept them.

iv. Grooming

Because of its short coat, the Italian Greyhound is a very easy dog to groom. Brushing only needs to be done about once a week, and it can be as easy as wiping them down with a damp cloth. This will remove the dead hair from the coat. Bathing should be done about once a month or whenever the dog needs it.

Nails should be trimmed monthly, and ears should be wiped clean whenever you wipe down the coat. Also, make sure that you brush the dog's teeth on a regular basis to prevent gum disease.

e) Health of the Breed

The average lifespan of the Italian Greyhound is between 12 to 15 years; however, over 16 years is not unheard of.

The breed is fairly healthy, but they do have some serious health problems potential owners should be aware of. It is important to do your research on this breed to ensure that you are purchasing from a line that is free of inherent diseases.

Health problems to be aware of with the Italian Greyhound are:

- Allergies
- Cataracts
- Cryptorchidism
- Epilepsy
- Hip Dysplasia
- Hypothyroidism
- Legg-Calve-Perthes Disease
- Patellar Luxation
- Portosystemic Shunt
- Progressive Retinal Atrophy
- Vitreous Degeneration
- Von Willebrand's Disease

f) Pros and Cons of the Breed

As you can imagine, there are a number of pros and cons to owning an Italian Greyhound, and it is important to weigh them before you bring one home.

Pros of the Italian Greyhound are:

- The small breed can live in any type of dwelling.

- They are known for being an elegant breed.

- While fast, the Italian Greyhound can be a couch potato, making it perfect for people who aren't overly active.

- They can also be quite active, so they can fit into an active lifestyle quite well.

- They are very easy to groom.

- The Italian Greyhound is known for being a quiet breed.

- They are usually affectionate with their owners and polite with everyone else.

- The breed is a low-shedding breed.

Cons of the Italian Greyhound are:

- The Italian Greyhound is a delicate breed and can be injured easily, which makes them better for homes without small children.

- They can be extremely shy, so socialization is a must.

- They are sensitive to changes in their schedule and can be affected by it greatly.

- The Italian Greyhound can become emotionally withdrawn when there is stress.

- Training can be difficult as the breed does have an independent nature.

- They have a high prey drive and are not recommended for homes with small pets.

- When outside, they should be leashed unless in a secure area.

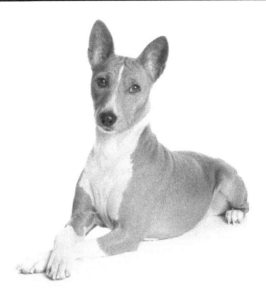

9. The Graceful Basenji

The Basenji is a small- to medium-sized dog that is known for being a quiet, cat-like breed. They are an exceptional family dog that is always ready to play. They love to lavish their owners with attention and are generally very good natured.

However, this is also a breed that does have an adventurous side so be prepared for some interesting adventures with your pup.

a) History of the Breed

Developed in West Africa, the Basenji is believed to be one of the oldest breeds alive today. In addition, the breed is believed to be one of the few primitive breeds around. The reason for this is that the breed maintains many characteristics seen in their wild cousins.

While they are an old breed, it is not clear how they were developed. What we do know is that the breed was used in the Congo region. Working with their human counterparts, the

Basenji would carry goods, flush game, or warn their humans to danger.

They were first discovered in the 1800s; however, attempts to bring the Basenji to Europe and North America failed for decades. This was due to the fact that the Basenji had never been exposed to certain diseases rampant in Europe, and any dogs imported would die from these diseases.

However, by the 1930s, several dogs were successfully imported into Europe and North America, and the breed quickly gained admirers. By 1942, the breed was established enough for the Basenji Club of America to be founded, and the breed was recognized by the AKC in 1943.

b) Temperament of the Breed

If there is one word that is used to describe the temperament of the Basenji, it is that they are cat-like. This is a breed that is very intelligent and alert.

They love being with their family and often do very well with children. They can be aloof with strangers and make excellent watchdogs as they will alert bark.

The breed has a very high prey drive, so they are not the best in homes with small animals. They are always eager to play and can make an excellent pet for active families.

One of the most interesting things to note with the Basenji is that they are very clean dogs and will actually groom themselves like a cat.

c) Appearance of the Breed

The Basenji is an athletic breed that should be sturdy and well-balanced. They should be graceful while still having a muscular build.

Basenjis should have a straight back with a body with straight legs. The tail should be carried high and should curl over the back of the dog.

The wedge-shaped head should be broad, and the muzzle should be short. There should be wrinkles on the forehead of the dog. Ears should be small and erect. They should face forward and give the dog an alert look.

i. Coat

The Basenji should have a very short coat. The single coat should be fine and should lay close to the dog's skin.

In coloration, the Basenji should have a striking appearance. They can be found in black, chestnut red, brindle, or tricolor with chestnut red, black, and white. All of the coat colors should have white markings. These markings should be on the tail tip, all four feet, and on the chest. White on the neck is also common as well as a blaze on the center of the dog's head, which is known as a blaze.

ii. Size

Basenjis are medium-sized dogs.

Height:
>   Males: 16 to 17 inches (40.6 to 43.2 cm)
>   Females: 15 to 16 inches (38.1 to 40.6cm)

Weight:
>   Males: 22 to 26 pounds (10 to 11.8kg)
>   Females: 20 to 25 pounds (9.1 to 11.3kg)

d) The Needs of the Breed

Basenjis, like all breeds, have specific needs that should be taken care of on a daily basis. This includes grooming, exercise, and training. Before you purchase a Basenji, make sure you understand the needs of the breed.

i. Exercise

The Basenji is an active breed, and they do need a lot of exercise. On average, your Basenji should receive about an hour to an hour and a half of exercise per day. They should not be trusted off leash when they are not in a secure area as they do like to wander.

In addition, they should not be trusted when they are in the yard. They do climb and will always find a way out of their yard if given the opportunity.

ii. Living Conditions

Although the breed does have a lot of energy, they can do well in apartments. The key is to give the Basenji a lot of exercise so they can live in apartments. They tend to only bark when necessary, so they usually aren't problem barkers.

The ideal setting for a Basenji is a home with a fenced yard so it can expel its energy.

iii. Ease of Training

The Basenji is a mixture of easy to train and difficult. On one hand, they do have a mind of their own so this can make them a challenge. Generally, training that becomes too repetitive or uses harsh correction will fail with the Basenji.

On the other hand, the Basenji is an eager-to-please breed, so if they find training fun and the owner provides clear and consistent rules, training can be easy.

They are naturally suspicious of strangers, so they need ample socialization to make them polite at the very least. In addition, owners should never trust a Basenji with a small, non-canine animal, even if they are well trained.

Finally, the Basenji is usually very easy to housetrain.

iv. Grooming Requirements

The Basenji is a very easy dog to groom. As I mentioned, they will groom themselves and stay fairly clean. Bathing should be done about once a month, if that, and brushing can simply be a wipe down with a wet cloth once a week.

Nails should be trimmed monthly, and ears should be wiped clean whenever you wipe down the coat.

e) Health of the Breed

The average lifespan of the Basenji is between 10 to 12 years.

They are considered to be a healthy breed; however, the Basenji does have a few health problems that can occur. It is important to do your research on this breed to ensure that you are purchasing from a line that is free of inherent diseases.

Health problems to be aware of with the Basenji are:

- Coloboma
- Fanconi Syndrome
- Hemolytic Anemia
- Hip Dysplasia
- Hypothyroidism
- Immunoproliferative Systemic Intestinal Disease
- Persistent Pupillary Membrane
- Progressive Retinal Atrophy
- Umbilical Hernia

f) Pros and Cons of the Breed

As you can imagine, there are a number of pros and cons to owning a Basenji, and it is important to weigh them before you bring one home.

Pros of the Basenji are:

- They are usually very easy to groom.

- The breed is a low-shedding breed, which makes it ideal for allergy sufferers.

- The breed can do well in most dwellings.

- They are affectionate with their family and do well with children.

- They make excellent watchdogs and will alert bark whenever they see something suspicious.

- The breed is easy to housetrain.

- They are active dogs that do well with an active family.

- They are very clean dogs.

- They are cat-like in temperament.

Cons of the Basenji are:

- They have high exercise requirements.

- The breed can be aggressive toward animals so socialization is a must.

- They have a high prey drive and may not be suitable in homes with small pets.

- The Basenji should be kept leashed when not in a secure area or they may chase other animals.

- They should not be left unattended in the yard as they will often try to run away.

- They can be destructive when they are bored.

- They can be difficult to train due to having a mind of their own.

- The Basenji is usually suspicious of strangers and will be aloof with new people.

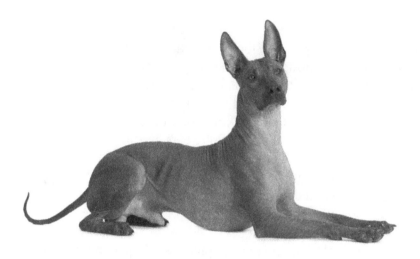

10. The Hairless Xoloitzcuintle

Pronounced so - low - EETs - kweenT - lee, the Xoloitzcuintle is a breed of dog that comes in a hairless variety, as well as a coated variety.

The breed is fairly unknown; however, it has quickly been gaining popularity, especially as a hypoallergenic breed. They do produce the allergen, but the lack of fur reduces the amount of irritants that come off of them.

This interesting breed is a wonderful companion that actually comes in several sizes. They are active, intelligent, and make wonderful companions for a range of lifestyles.

a) History of the Breed

Also known as the Mexican Hairless, the Xoloitzcuintle is believed to be one of the oldest breeds that are alive today. While it is unclear when the breed was developed, depictions of the breed can be dated back to 3,000 years ago. In fact, the breed is believed to have been prized as mystical creatures by the Mayan, Colima, and also the Aztec.

While we know where the breed originated, it is unclear how the breed was developed. It is believed that the first people who crossed the land bridge from Asia to the Americas brought with them a hairless dog that was called a "Biche." It is believed that these hairless dogs developed into what we see today; however, it is interesting to note that the Xoloitzcuintle is relatively unchanged from what it was 3,000 years ago.

During the 1800s, the breed was close to extinction; however, interest in the breed during the 1900s helped the breed build its numbers again.

Today, the Xoloitzcuintle is a popular family pet and has proven itself as a versatile breed.

b) Temperament of the Breed

The Xoloitzcuintle breed is known for being a very intelligent breed that does well with just about anyone. They are excellent as family dogs as they are very loving to their people. They love children and are usually very patient with them.

In addition to being loving and intelligent, this is an athletic breed that thrives in homes of active families. They can make excellent jogging companions and are always willing to go and do something with their owners.

That being said, this is a breed that will try to run away if the opportunity presents itself. They are amazing escape artists and will climb, dig, and even jump to get out of a yard. It is important that you never leave them unattended in the yard and to keep them leashed when they are out of the yard.

When it comes to strangers, the Xoloitzcuintle is not overly friendly. They are naturally suspicious of people and are excellent watchdogs. When they are properly trained and socialized, the

Xoloitzcuintle can be a polite dog to people outside of its family, but it does not adjust to change readily.

The breed can be strong willed, so it is important to be firm and consistent with training and rules.

c) Appearance of the Breed

The Xoloitzcuintle is a small- to medium-sized dog that should have an athletic build. The body should be slightly longer than it is tall, and it should have a robust appearance.

The head should be wedge-shaped with a broad skull and medium length muzzle. The ears are often the most noticeable of the Xoloitzcuintle's appearance. They should be large and erect and resemble bat ears.

i. Coat

The Xoloitzcuintle has two different coats, and both are considered hypoallergenic. The one that is more commonly seen is the hairless variety. They are usually completely hairless, but some may have hair on the top of their head, the tip of their tail, and also on the feet.

The haired variety, or coated, should have a short, single layer coat that fits close to the skin. The coat should be smooth to the touch.

In regards to coloring, all colors are accepted, and it is seen on the skin as well. Xoloitzcuintle can be red, gray, gray-black, black, liver, slate, or bronze. White markings are also very common with all the colors.

ii. Size

There are three different sizes for the Xoloitzcuintle; however, all three sizes have the same structure, temperament, and needs. The sizes are:

Toy:
9 to 14 inches (22.9 to 35.6cm) in height
5 to 15 pounds (2.3 to 6.8kg) in weight

Miniature:
15 to 20 inches (38.1 to 50.8cm) in height
15 to 30 pounds (6.8 to 13.6kg) in weight

Standard:
20 to 30 inches (50.8 to 76.2cm) or more in height
30 to 60 pounds (13.6 to 27.2kg) in weight

d) The Needs of the Breed

Xoloitzcuintles, like all breeds, have specific needs that should be taken care of on a daily basis. This includes grooming, exercise, and training. Before you purchase a Xoloitzcuintle, make sure you understand the needs of the breed.

i. Exercise

Regardless of the size of Xoloitzcuintle that you have, you should be prepared for the exercise needs of this dog. Even the smaller Xoloitzcuintle will need a 30-minute walk every day while the larger Xoloitzcuintle will require about an hour.

Remember that the Xoloitzcuintle is hairless, so whenever you exercise your dog, make sure it's dressed for the weather.

ii. Living Conditions

Xoloitzcuintle can do well in any setting and can do very well in apartments as long as they are getting daily exercise.

iii. Ease of Training

The Xoloitzcuintle can be a difficult breed to train because they have a mind of their own. This breed is very intelligent, and they can become bored with repetitive training.

In addition, the Xoloitzcuintle is a sensitive breed, and any harsh corrections can shut them down. They should only be trained with positive reinforcement so they stay happy during the training and do not shut down.

Socialization is a must with the Xoloitzcuintle as they can be very suspicious of strangers. They usually do well with other animals, but it is important to get them out and around people.

One thing that should be highlighted with the Xoloitzcuintle is that they are very challenging when they are young. They need lots of training and socialization, and they need to spend a lot of time with their owners for bonding. If you do not pay a lot of attention to this breed while they are young, you will have problems later on in their life.

iv. Grooming Requirements

Despite having very little hair, the Xoloitzcuintle is a breed that has a lot of grooming requirements, and it usually falls into skin care.

In general, you should avoid over-bathing the breed and should only bathe them once or twice a year. In addition, make sure that you apply oil on their skin after bathing to keep them from developing dry skin.

Use sunscreen when you are taking your Xoloitzcuintle outside and during the warmer months. Make sure you wipe off the excess sunscreen at the end of the day as too much product can clog the pores of your Xoloitzcuintle and cause skin problems.

Finally, you will need to treat acne from time to time, but make sure you use an exfoliating scrub instead of an acne medication.

As with all dogs, teeth should be brushed regularly, and the nails should be trimmed about once or twice a month.

e) Health of the Breed

The average lifespan of the Xoloitzcuintle is between 14 to 15 years, although some lines have reached 20 years of age.

The Xoloitzcuintle is a very hardy breed, and currently, there are no known health problems in the breed. They do have sensitive skin, so it is important to provide them with proper skin care to prevent injury. Other than that, the breed has very few health problems.

f) Pros and Cons of the Breed

As you can imagine, there are a number of pros and cons to owning a Xoloitzcuintle, and it is important to weigh them before you bring one home.

Pros of the Xoloitzcuintle are:

- They can do well in a range of dwellings.

- They are very agile dogs that can be a joy to watch.

- The Xoloitzcuintle is a breed that is very smart.

- They are canine acrobats and will jump, climb, and run.

- They are perfect dogs for an active family.

- They do well with older children.

- They can be found in several sizes.

- They are hairless, so they are a non-shedding breed.

- They do well with other animals.

- They are a very intelligent breed.

Cons of the Xoloitzcuintle are:

- They thrive when they are with their owners and can suffer from separation anxiety.

- They can be very timid and are usually suspicious of strangers. Socialization is a must with this breed.

- They can be difficult to train since they have a mind of their own.

- Xoloitzcuintle can be problem barkers.

- The breed has high grooming needs to help protect its skin.

- The Xoloitzcuintle will try to escape from yards, so they should be monitored when outside.

- They can be difficult to housetrain.

- The breed is very sensitive and can become stressed very easily.

Chapter Five: Top 5 Hypoallergenic Cross Breeds

Now that we have gone over some of the popular purebred dogs that are hypoallergenic, it is time to go over some of the cross breeds. The crossbreeds in this chapter are breeds that do very well with allergy sufferers.

Like their purebred counterparts, these crossbreeds are dogs that either produce small amounts of the protein allergen or they produce very little hair. Both qualities help in them being hypoallergenic.

Like I did with the purebred breeds, I will take you through each breed. This will include going over the size, temperament, and history of the breed, as well as the health problems that each breed has. I will also take you through the pros and cons of the breed and all the other information you will need.

By the end of each breed profile, you should have a clear understanding of the breed and whether it will fit into your home and lifestyle.

As I have mentioned, this chapter is on crossbreeds, which are also known as designer breeds, which is where two dog breeds have been bred together to create a new breed. Many times, there is a trait that breeders are trying to produce with this crossing.

The difference between a crossbreed and a purebred is that with a crossbreed, the parents are from two separate breeds, and with a purebred, the parents are from the same. With that explanation, let's get started.

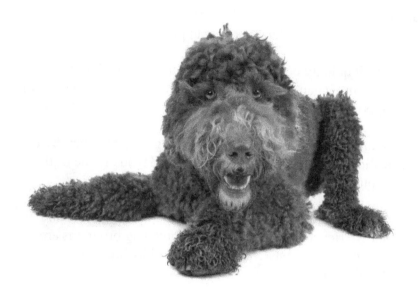

1. The Silly Labradoodle

The Labradoodle is a happy companion that does well in a variety of homes. They are usually very loving and are actually the most popular crossbreed around.

The breed has shown itself to be intelligent, loyal, and an all around versatile dog.

a) History of the Breed

The Labradoodle has the distinction of being one of the first designer breeds. Originally, the breed was developed in an effort to create a hypoallergenic guide dog.

Developed in Australia by the Royal Guide Dog Association and Wally Conron in 1989, the Labradoodle was created by crossing the Poodle with the Labrador Retriever.

The very first breedings of the Labradoodle produced a dog named Sultan. The dog was a hypoallergenic dog with all of the traits needed for a guide dog. His work as a guide dog drew the interest of several breeders who began producing their own dogs.

However, it quickly became apparent that the Labradoodle was a failed crossing when it came to the guide dog work and also with being hypoallergenic as only certain coats were hypoallergenic.

Wally Conron abandoned the breeding program; however, by the time he did, enough interest in the breed had made it one of the more popular dog breeds around.

While you can still purchase a Labradoodle with a Poodle and Labrador Retriever parent, many of the breeding programs are starting to create a consistent breed standard by breeding Labradoodle to Labradoodle.

b) Temperament of the Breed

An intelligent breed, the Labradoodle is a friendly dog that generally gets along with everyone. They are usually an excellent family dog as they do well with children of all ages.

The breed is very energetic and needs to have outlets, both intellectually and physically. When they are exercised properly, they tend to be very laid back and easy going. They can be natural clowns and love to play.

c) Appearance of the Breed

The Labradoodle ranges in size from small to large and is the result of crossing the Labrador Retriever with the Poodle. The size of the dog greatly depends on the variety of Poodle used in the crossing.

The breed should have a slightly rectangular shape with the length being slightly longer than the height. They should have a level back and should have the appearance of an athletic dog. The Labradoodle should have a broad head with a long muzzle. They should have a slightly rounded skull, like their poodle parent, but the wider muzzle of the lab.

Ears of the Labradoodle should be long and hanging. They should be kept close to the head. They should never be carried high and should never be cropped. The tail should be medium in length and carried high.

i. Coat

The coat of the Labradoodle varies depending on the parent that the dog takes after. There are actually three coat types that you can see. The hair coat is usually a straighter coat that has a thick undercoat. It is usually about four to six inches in length; however, it can be longer. This coat sheds the most out of all the coat types.

The fleece coat is another shedding coat, although it is a low-shedding coat that can range in texture from straight to wavy. This coat has a soft undercoat and a heavy, silky-to-the-touch top coat.

The wool coat, which is the most desired, is non-shedding and has a wool-like texture. The coat has a dense undercoat and a curly topcoat.

Labradoodles can be any color, but the most common are apricot, black, white, blue, chalk, silver, gold, parchment, chocolate, cafe, red, caramel, and cream. They can also be parti-colored with black and white, red and white, grey and white, or any other combination with white. They can also have brindles, patched, sable, or phantom coloration.

ii. Size

There are three different sizes for the Labradoodle; however, all three sizes have the same structure, temperament, and needs. The sizes are:

Toy:

> 14 to 17 inches (35.7 to 43.2cm) in height
> 10 to 25 pounds (4.5 to 11.3kg) in weight

Miniature:

> 17 to 20 inches (43.2 to 50.8cm) in height
> 25 to 45 pounds (11.3 to 20.4kg) in weight

Standard:

> 20 to 24 inches (43.2 to 60.1cm) or more in height
> 45 to 100 pounds (20.4 to 45.3kg) in weight

d) The Needs of the Breed

Labradoodles, like all breeds, have specific needs that should be taken care of on a daily basis. This includes grooming, exercise, and training. Before you purchase a Labradoodle, make sure you understand the needs of the breed.

i. Exercise

The Labradoodle is an energetic breed and requires a large amount of exercise every day. Expect to give the dog about one hour of exercise. The breed can do very well as jogging companions.

In addition to physical exercise, make sure that you give the dog plenty of intellectual stimulation. This is an intelligent breed that needs to be properly stimulated or they will become destructive.

ii. Living Conditions

Although a well-exercised Labradoodle can do okay in an apartment, the ideal living condition is a home with a fenced yard. The breed does very well with other animals and pets and is an excellent family dog.

iii. Ease of Training

Training can vary depending on whether the dog takes after their Poodle parent or Labrador Retriever parent. Usually, they are an eager-to-please dog that is very food-motivated. The occasional Labradoodle can have a mind of its own, but having clear and consistent rules will help with training.

Socialization is a must for a Labradoodle so they can learn how to behave in public.

iv. Grooming Requirements

Labradoodles, regardless of coat type, should be groomed every other day or several times a week. This will help keep hair to a minimum. You can trim the coat to make it more manageable; however, if you trim it, it should be clipped every 4 to 6 weeks.

Bathing should be done about once per month and only when necessary. Ears should be cleaned weekly since the breed can be prone to ear infections. Teeth should be brushed weekly, and nails should be clipped monthly.

e) Health of the Breed

The average lifespan of the Labradoodle is between 12 to 14 years.

It is important to note that crossbreed dogs are considered to have what is called hybrid vigor, which means they are healthier. However, this vigor is usually seen in second and third generations and not first generation crosses. In addition, if the parents carry inherent diseases, then they can pass them on to their young, regardless of whether they are purebred or crossbred.

Labradoodles themselves are considered to be a healthy breed; however, the breed does have a few health problems that can occur. It is important to do your research on this breed to ensure that you are purchasing from a line that is free of inherent diseases.

Health problems to be aware of with the Labradoodle are:

- Allergies
- Diabetes Mellitus
- Ear Infections
- Elbow Dysplasia
- Epilepsy
- Hip Dysplasia
- Hypothyroidism
- Progressive Retinal Atrophy

f) Pros and Cons of the Breed

As you can imagine, there are a number of pros and cons to owning a Labradoodle, and it is important to weigh them before you bring one home.

Pros of the Labradoodle are:

- The breed can be found in varying sizes, making it a versatile breed that can fit into any lifestyle.

- They make excellent jogging companions because of their energy.

- The breed is an excellent family dog that does well with children.

- They usually get along well with everyone; however, they will alert bark.

- The breed is usually easy to train.

- The Labradoodle is usually good with other animals.

- They can be very goofy and are a joy to live with.

- Efforts are being made to create a breed standard with the Labradoodle, which will help establish ethical breeding.

- The easy nature of the Labradoodle makes them perfect for first-time dog owners.

Cons of the Labradoodle are:

- They are a popular breed for puppy mills and backyard breeders, so it is important to research your breeder.

- The breed is very energetic and needs a lot of exercise.

- They can have energetic behaviors such as jumping and being rambunctious.

- Not all Labradoodles are hypoallergenic. The coat type is an important factor in this. The curly and wavy coat type, which is closer to the Poodle coat than the Labrador Retriever's, is more likely to be hypoallergenic.

- The breed is not the best choice for an apartment; however, they can live in one with ample exercise.

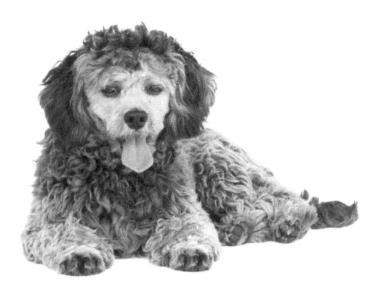

2. The Cuddly Shih Poo

The Shih Poo is a little teddy bear that is quickly capturing the hearts of dog fanciers everywhere. The breed is known for being an affectionate crossbreed that loves spending time with its family. In fact, the Shih Poo is just as happy spending the day perched on the lap as it is getting out for a walk.

a) History of the Breed

The history of the Shih Poo is not as in-depth as other crosses. It was simply created when the popularity of Poodle crosses was at its peak. It was developed in an effort to create a companion dog that had the temperament of the Shih Tzu but the coat of the Poodle.

b) Temperament of the Breed

The Shih Poo is a sweet little dog that is known for being a friendly companion. Generally, the breed gets along well with everyone, and they are very affectionate with their owners.

They can be quite playful. The breed is known for being intelligent, and they love to do tricks for their owners. Overall, the Shih Poo is an excellent companion dog for families or older couples.

c) Appearance of the Breed

The Shih Poo is a cute, teddy bear-like dog that has a slightly longer body than it is tall. It should be robust with a graceful gait, and it should have a broad head. The ears should be long and hang down the sides of the head. The muzzle should be short like the Shih Tzu, but the head should be rounded like the Poodle.

i. Coat

The coat of the Shih Poo will vary depending on the parent they take after. It may be long and thick or curly and dense. All of the coat varieties have a double coat, with a soft, short undercoat and a longer top coat.

They can be any color, including black, white, gray, brown, gold, apricot, and red. They can also be parti-colored or be white with colored markings.

ii. Size

The Shih Poo is a toy- to small-sized breed of dog. Males and females have roughly the same size.

Height
8 to 15 inches (20.3 to 38.1cm)

Weight
>7 to 20 pounds (3.2 to 9.1kg)

d) The Needs of the Breed

Shih Poos, like all breeds, have specific needs that should be taken care of on a daily basis. This includes grooming, exercise, and training. Before you purchase a Shih Poo, make sure you understand the needs of the breed.

i. Exercise

Although the Shih Poo is an energetic breed, the small size makes it very easy for the breed to be exercised. Even a game in the house can help them expel their energy.

Still, the breed should have about 30 minutes of exercise per day outside. If you keep them in the yard, make sure you monitor them as they can be injured by larger animals.

ii. Living Conditions

The Shih Poo does amazing in any type of dwelling and is a perfect apartment companion. They can do well in homes with other animals as well as homes with children. It should be noted that their small size makes them better suited to homes with older children.

iii. Ease of Training

The Shih Poo can be easy to train since it is an intelligent breed; however, it can have a stubborn streak from time to time. It is important to give firm rules to make training easier.

Owners should avoid babying the breed as they can suffer from Small Dog Syndrome. When this occurs, you may have to deal with destructive behavior, problem barking, and a host of other problems.

To avoid Small Dog Syndrome, place firm and consistent rules in the house. Socialization should be done with the Shih Poo, but they usually get along well with everyone.

iv. Grooming Requirements

The Shih Poo, like many of the Poodle crosses, has varying needs when it comes to grooming. These requirements are dependent on the type of coat the dog inherited.

With the Shih Poo, most owners opt to keep the coat short to make grooming easier. This means the dog should be clipped every 4 to 6 weeks or whenever the hair grows long. Even with clipping, the coat should be brushed weekly.

Bathing should be done when the coat is clipped. If you keep the coat long, it should be bathed weekly and brushed daily.

If the Shih Poo has the same eye structure as its Shih Tzu parent, take the time to wash the eyes weekly. Administer drops to keep the eyes from drying out, but only under the recommendations of your vet. Finally, make sure that you trim the nails on a monthly basis.

e) Health of the Breed

The average lifespan of the Shih Poo is between 14 to 15 years; however, it is not uncommon for Shih Poos to live longer than 15 years.

It is important to note that crossbreed dogs are considered to have what is called hybrid vigor, which means they are healthier. However, this vigor is usually seen in second and third generations and not first generation crosses. In addition, if the parents carry inherent diseases, then they can pass them on to their young, regardless of whether they are purebred or crossbred.

Shih Poos themselves are considered to be a healthy breed; however, the breed does have a few health problems that can occur. It is important to do your research on this breed to ensure that you are purchasing from a line that is free of inherent diseases.

Health problems to be aware of with the Shih Poo are:

- Addison's Disease
- Allergies
- Bladder Infections
- Bladder Stones
- Bloat, also known as Gastric Dilatation-Volvulus
- Cataracts
- Cushing's Disease, also known as Hyperadrenocorticism
- Diabetes
- Distichiasis
- Ear Infections
- Ectopia Cilia
- Epilepsy
- Gum Disease
- Heart Disease
- Hip Dysplasia
- Hypothyroidism
- Immune Mediated Hemolytic Anemia
- Juvenile Renal Dysplasia
- Keratitis
- Keratoconjunctivitis Sicca
- Legg-Perthes Disease
- Optic Nerve Hypoplasia
- Patellar Luxation
- Portosystemic Liver Shunt
- Progressive Retinal Atrophy
- Proptosis
- Retained Baby Teeth
- Reverse Sneezing
- Sebaceous Adenitis

- Slipped Stifle
- Snuffles
- Umbilical Hernia
- Van Willebrand's Disease

f) Pros and Cons of the Breed

As you can imagine, there are a number of pros and cons to owning a Shih Poo, and it is important to weigh them before you bring one home.

Pros of the Shih Poo are:

- They are excellent companions for people who live in apartments.

- The breed is usually quite friendly and loyal.

- The Shih Poo is a small dog that can and will go everywhere.

- They do well with older children.

- The breed has lower exercise needs.

- They are very loyal to their owners.

- The Shih Poo is usually very easy to train.

Cons of the Shih Poo are:

- They are another popular breed with puppy mills, so make sure you research the breeder.

- They can be difficult to groom.

- The Shih Poo is a small breed and can suffer from Small Dog Syndrome, which can lead to many behavior problems.

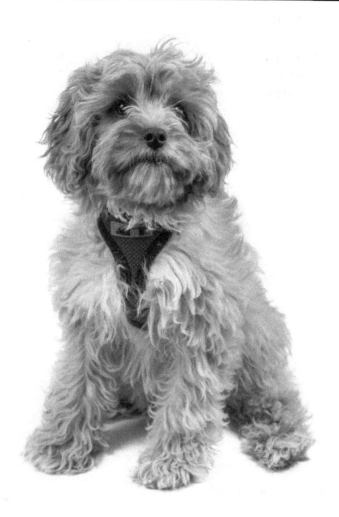

3. The Charming Cavapoo

The charming Cavapoo is exactly that: charming. They are known for being an affectionate breed that loves nothing more than simply being with their owners. They are excellent family dogs, and their robust build, affectionate temperament, and friendly disposition makes them ideal for families with children.

a) History of the Breed

Another of the older crossbreeds, the Cavapoo was first seen in the United States in the 1950s. It was developed by crossing the Cavalier King Charles Spaniel and the Toy Poodle. The breed was created in an attempt to make a non-shedding breed with many of the qualities of the Cavalier King Charles Spaniel.

The breed was very successful, and it is one of the more popular designer breeds that are being produced. Many breeders are currently breeding Cavapoo to Cavapoo in an effort to create a breed standard. However, the main focus of breeding is to create a hypoallergenic family dog that has few health problems.

b) Temperament of the Breed

Affectionate and loyal are two words that are commonly used to describe this breed. They are generally very friendly dogs that are naturally charming. This is a breed that really does get along with everyone, and they thrive when they can be social.

In fact, the Cavapoo does not like to be alone and prefer to be with their owners. The robust breed can do very well with children of all ages. In addition, the breed is very good with other pets.

c) Appearance of the Breed

The Cavapoo is a fluffy little teddy bear of a dog with a slightly rectangular body. It should have a sturdy appearance and should not be delicate at all, despite its small size. The top line of the dog should be level and straight, and it should have a medium-long tail.

The head of the Cavapoo is slightly rounded and broad. The muzzle should be thick and medium in length. Ears should be long and hang down the side of the head. Their face should be very expressive.

i. Coat

Cavapoos have a range of coat types from very tight curls like the Poodle to the long wavy locks of the Cavalier King Charles Spaniel. The preferred coat for the Cavapoo is a soft curl that is closer to the Poodle parent.

Colors of the breed include white, black and white, brown and white, gold, and finally, black, white, and tan.

ii. Size

The Cavapoo is a toy- to small-sized breed of dog. Males and females have roughly the same size.

Height
9 to 14 inches (22.9 to 35.6cm)

Weight
7 to 18 pounds (3.2 to 8.2kg)

d) The Needs of the Breed

Cavapoos, like all breeds, have specific needs that should be taken care of on a daily basis. This includes grooming, exercise, and training. Before you purchase a Cavapoo, make sure you understand the needs of the breed.

i. Exercise

The exercise requirements of the Cavapoo are actually fairly easy to meet. They will often expel their energy with a good game of fetch in the house, but usually a 15 to 20 minute walk per day is all the exercise they need.

ii. Living Conditions

Cavapoos are versatile breeds that can do very well in a range of dwellings. Their small size and low exercise needs makes them ideal pets for apartments.

One word of caution is that Cavapoos can become problem barkers, so make sure that your building does not have noise restrictions.

iii. Ease of Training

The Cavapoo is an intelligent breed that can be easy to train if positive reinforcement is used. They can be sensitive, so avoid any type of harsh correction with them.

As with all small dogs, avoid carrying them around and babying them. This can lead to Small Dog Syndrome, which can lead to destructive behavior and other problems.

iv. Grooming Requirements

The Cavapoo has grooming requirements that can differ slightly depending on the coat type. Generally, all coat types should be brushed every few days to prevent matting. In addition, the coat should be trimmed every 6 to 8 weeks so the dog continues to have a tidy appearance.

Ears should be cleaned weekly, and it is important to check them regularly as the breed can be prone to ear infections. The Cavapoo should have its nails trimmed about once a month.

Finally, check and clean the Cavapoo's eyes regularly as they can be prone to eye problems, including dry eye.

e) Health of the Breed

The average lifespan of the Cavapoo is between 10 to 15 years.

It is important to note that crossbreed dogs are considered to have what is called hybrid vigor, which means they are healthier. However, this vigor is usually seen in second and third generations and not first generation crosses. In addition, if the parents carry inherent diseases, then they can pass them on to their young, regardless of whether they are purebred or crossbred.

Cavapoos themselves are considered to be a healthy breed; however, the breed does have a few health problems that can occur. It is important to do your research on this breed to ensure that you are purchasing from a line that is free of inherent diseases.

Health problems to be aware of with the Cavapoo are:

- Addison's Disease
- Bloat; also known as hypoadrenocorticism
- Cushing's Disease
- Epilepsy
- Episodic Falling
- Hip Dysplasia
- Hypothyroidism
- Keratoconjunctivitis Sicca
- Legg-Perthes Disease
- Mitral Valve Disease
- Patellar Luxation
- Progressive Retinal Atrophy
- Optic Nerve Hypoplasia
- Sebaceous Adenitis
- Syringomyelia
- Von Willebrand's Disease

f) Pros and Cons of the Breed

As you can imagine, there are a number of pros and cons to owning a Cavapoo, and it is important to weigh them before you bring one home.

Pros of the Cavapoo are:

- The breed is versatile and can live just about anywhere.

- They are known for being very friendly.

- The Cavapoo does very well with children of all ages.

- They are loyal to their owners.

- They are low-shedding.

- They are usually easy to train.

- The breed has a lower exercise requirement.

Cons of the Cavapoo are:

- It is another popular breed with puppy mills, so make sure you research the breeder.

- The Cavapoo is a small breed and can suffer from Small Dog Syndrome, which can lead to many behavior problems.

- The breed thrives with their owners, so they can suffer from separation anxiety when they are away from them.

- The Cavapoo can be a problem barker.

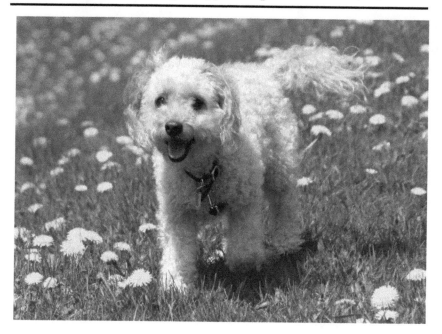

4. The Affectionate Cockapoo

One of the oldest and most loved crossbreeds, the Cockapoo is the result of crossing the Cocker Spaniel and the Poodle. The result is a compact companion dog that is affectionate, loyal, and above all else...happy.

a) History of the Breed

Although the Cockapoo is a designer breed, it is one of the oldest designer breeds around. Originally developed in the 1960s, it is believed that the first pairing was completely accidental. However, when the puppies produced had an amazing temperament and a hypoallergenic coat, breeders realized that they were an excellent breed.

This led to many breeders producing the Cockapoo. In addition, the breeders are serious in making the Cockapoo a fully recognized breed with Kennel Clubs. Efforts have been made to create multigenerational lines, and the Cockapoo Club of America has been established since 1999.

Today, breeders are moving toward getting the Cockapoo recognized and continue to breed toward a standard.

b) Temperament of the Breed

Happy, intelligent, and a gentle dog that is friendly to everyone, the Cockapoo is known for its outgoing temperament. The breed is usually very calm; however, some can be problem barkers.

The breed is very intelligent, and they will happily perform tricks for their owners. They do well in busy homes with older children and animals. The breed is outgoing, but they do not have too much energy. They are always happy to snuggle with their owners.

c) Appearance of the Breed

A small-sized dog, the Cockapoo actually takes after the Cocker Spaniel parent when it comes to shape and look. They are usually a robust dog that has a sturdy appearance. The head is slightly rounded while the muzzle is short and thick. The ears should hang down the side of the head, and the tail often curls over the back of the dog.

i. Coat

The Cockapoo can have a variety of coats, and it really depends on what parent breed they take after. The most common coat is a wavy double coat that has a thick undercoat and a moderately long topcoat. However, the coat can be curly like a Poodle or long and silky like a Cocker Spaniel.

Cockapoos can be any color, including black, brown, cream, red, apricot, buff, white, sable, auburn, beige, brindle, silver, and roan. Many of them are white with colored markings, but you can find solids or colors with white markings.

ii. Size

Cockapoos are a toy- to small-sized breed of dog. Males and females have roughly the same size.

Height
>   10 to 15 inches (30.5 to 38.1cm)

Weight
>   12 to 24 pounds (5.4 to 10.9kg)

d) The Needs of the Breed

Cockapoos, like all breeds, have specific needs that should be taken care of on a daily basis. This includes grooming, exercise, and training. Before you purchase a Cockapoo, make sure you understand the needs of the breed.

i. Exercise

The Cockapoo is a breed that does not require a lot of exercise. Usually 15 to 20 minutes of exercise is enough to meet their needs.

That being said, this is a breed that can do very well in dog sports such as agility. They also love to swim, so make sure you give your Cockapoo a range of activities to do.

ii. Living Conditions

Cockapoos can do very well in apartments and are a versatile breed. They can also do well in homes with lots of other pets and also in homes with children.

iii. Ease of Training

Overall, the Cockapoo is an easy breed to train. They are usually eager to please and they tend to be very intelligent. Housetraining can take a bit longer than other breeds, but it really depends on the consistency of the owner.

Owners should avoid babying the breed as they can suffer from Small Dog Syndrome. When this occurs, you may have to deal with destructive behavior, problem barking, and a host of other problems.

To avoid Small Dog Syndrome, place firm and consistent rules in the house. Socialization should be done with the Cockapoo, but they usually get along well with everyone.

iv. Grooming Requirements

Grooming requirements differ depending on the coat type of the breed. Most of the dogs need to be brushed on a daily basis to keep the coat free of mats. This is very important if the dog is kept in full coat. However, to make it easier, many owners clip the dog's coat short. Clipping should be done every 4 to 6 weeks and should be all over the body of the dog.

In addition to clipping, bathing should be done weekly with the Cockapoo in full coat or about once a month when the coat is clipped. Teeth should be brushed weekly, nails should be clipped monthly, and the ears should be cleaned whenever the teeth are brushed.

e) Health of the Breed

The average lifespan of the Cockapoo is between 12 to 15 years.

It is important to note that crossbreed dogs are considered to have what is called hybrid vigor, which means they are healthier. However, this vigor is usually seen in second and third generations and not first generation crosses. In addition, if the parents carry inherent diseases, then they can pass them on to their young, regardless of whether they are purebred or crossbred.

Cockapoos themselves are considered to be a healthy breed; however, the breed does have a few health problems that can occur. It is important to do your research on this breed to ensure that you are purchasing from a line that is free of inherent diseases.

Health problems to be aware of with the Cockapoo are:

- Allergies
- Cataracts
- Ear Infections
- Hip Dysplasia
- Liver Disease
- Patellar Luxation

f) Pros and Cons of the Breed

As you can imagine, there are a number of pros and cons to owning a Cockapoo, and it is important to weigh them before you bring one home.

Pros of the Cockapoo are:

- The breed is versatile and can live just about anywhere.

- They are known for being very friendly.

- They are low-shedding.

- They are usually easy to train.

- They do very well with children.

- The Cockapoo has a lower exercise requirement.

Cons of the Cockapoo are:

- It is another popular breed with puppy mills, so make sure you research the breeder.

- They can be difficult to groom.

- The Cockapoo is a small breed and can suffer from Small Dog Syndrome, which can lead to many behavior problems.

- They can be problem barkers.

- They can be slow to housetrain.

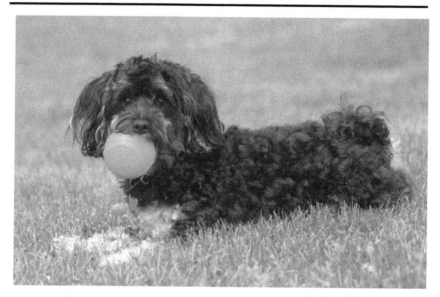

5. The Cute Maltipoo

The Maltipoo is a fairly new breed that has gained popularity since the start of the designer dog craze. It is a sweet dog with a delicate appearance and a very happy and affectionate nature. This is a true companion breed that loves being with their owners.

a) History of the Breed

The history of the Maltipoo is quite short since the breed is a fairly new breed. It became a popular breed in the 1990s to early 2000s when designer breeds became popular.

The Maltipoo was developed by crossing the Maltese with the Toy Poodle. The result was a companion breed with a long, hypoallergenic coat. While some breeders are making an effort to establish a breed standard, the Maltipoo has not been established yet.

b) Temperament of the Breed

Known for being a funny and affectionate dog, the Maltipoo often captures the hearts of anyone they meet. They are very loyal to their owners and are completely devoted to them. They tend to have a feisty nature, and while they are friendly, the breed is usually protective of their owners. They can be suspicious of strangers, and this makes them wonderful watchdogs.

The breed is usually very gentle; however, their small size does not make them a good match for children. The breed can be quite active, but it doesn't take much exercise to tire them out.

c) Appearance of the Breed

Maltipoos are a toy-sized breed that should be delicate and graceful. The slightly square dog should have a straight and level back. The head should be slightly rounded with a delicate muzzle. Ears should hang down and should lie close to the head. The tail should be medium in length.

i. Coat

As with all the crossbreeds, the coat of the Maltipoo can range from the silky coat of the Maltese to the curly coat of the Poodle. However, the most common coat type of the Maltipoo is the wool-like coat. This coat is usually medium in length and has a slight wave to a soft curl. The coat should be fluffy and should be low-shedding.

The Maltipoo can be found in all of the colors; however, the most common, and desired, are silver, cream, and white.

ii. Size

The Maltipoo is a toy-sized breed of dog. Males and females have roughly the same size.

Height
> 7 to 14 inches (17.8 to 35.6cm)

Weight
> 10 to 15 pounds (4.5 to 6.8kg)

d) The Needs of the Breed

Maltipoos, like all breeds, have specific needs that should be taken care of on a daily basis. This includes grooming, exercise, and training. Before you purchase a Maltipoo, make sure you understand the needs of the breed.

i. Exercise

The exercise requirements of the Maltipoo are actually fairly easy to meet. They will often expel their energy with a good game of fetch in the house, but usually a 15 to 20 minute walk per day is all the exercise they need.

ii. Living Conditions

Another versatile breed, the Maltipoo can live in any type of dwelling. They do very well in apartments, but again, like many small breeds, they can be problem barkers.

iii. Ease of Training

When it comes to training, the Maltipoo is average with ease. They can be easy to train if they find training interesting; however, they can have a stubborn streak that makes training difficult.

Owners should provide clear and consistent rules. In addition, they should use positive reinforcement with this breed. The Maltipoo can suffer from Small Dog Syndrome, so make sure that you do not baby them.

iv. Grooming Requirements

The coat of the Maltipoo can be fairly easy to groom. It requires daily brushing to keep it free from mats, but this should only take a few minutes a day. The breed should be bathed about once a month to keep the coat in top condition.

Eyes should be kept clean, as should the ears. It may be necessary to trim the hair in the ears and around the eyes to keep the dog tidy. Nails should be clipped monthly.

e) Health of the Breed

The average lifespan of the Maltipoo is between 10 to 13 years.

It is important to note that crossbreed dogs are considered to have what is called hybrid vigor, which means they are healthier. However, this vigor is usually seen in second and third generations and not first generation crosses. In addition, if the parents carry inherent diseases, then they can pass them on to their young, regardless of whether they are purebred or crossbred.

Maltipoos themselves are considered to be a healthy breed; however, the breed does have a few health problems that can occur. It is important to do your research on this breed to ensure that you are purchasing from a line that is free of inherent diseases.

Health problems to be aware of with the Maltipoo are:

- Epilepsy
- Legg-Calve-Perthes Disease
- Patellar Luxation
- Portosystemic Shunt
- Progressive Retinal Atrophy
- White Shaker Syndrome

f) Pros and Cons of the Breed

As you can imagine, there are a number of pros and cons to owning a Maltipoo, and it is important to weigh them before you bring one home.

Pros of the Maltipoo are:

- They are fiercely devoted to their owners.

- They make excellent watchdogs as they will alert bark.

- The coat is low-shedding, making them excellent for allergy sufferers.

- The breed does very well in apartments.

- The breed has a lower exercise requirement.

Cons of the Maltipoo are:

- It is another popular breed with puppy mills, so make sure you research the breeder.

- The breed can suffer from separation anxiety, which can lead to destructive behavior.

- They are not a good match with children.

- The Maltipoo can have problems housetraining.

- The Maltipoo is a small breed and can suffer from Small Dog Syndrome, which can lead to many behavior problems, including becoming a problem barker.

- The breed thrives with their owners, so they can suffer from separation anxiety when they are away from them.

Chapter Six: Frequently Asked Questions

Hopefully I have answered all the questions that you have regarding your hypoallergenic dog, but before I end this book with some valuable resources, I want to take the time to answer some frequently asked questions. This is just in case I missed anything in the book.

1. FAQ about Allergies

What is an allergy?

An allergy is when a person or animal, yes even dogs can have allergies, has an abnormally high sensitivity to a substance, known as an allergen. The immune system of the allergy sufferers views this substance as an invader and produces a reaction to it as it tries to combat the foreign substance with antibodies.

What are the most common allergens?

Allergies are different for everyone, but in general, the top allergens are:

- Animal produced proteins, often found in dander
- Dust
- Mold
- Pollen
- Peanuts
- Latex
- Eggs

How do I know if I or someone I love has allergies?

It is often very easy to identify that you or someone in your home has allergies. Itchy eyes, sneezing, sinuses filling up, rashes, and hives are all common symptoms.

That being said, it is important to be diagnosed by an allergist to ensure that you pinpoint the reason for your allergy. Many times, the allergen trigger may not even be pets, although it may seem like it is.

How can you tell the difference between allergies and a cold?

If you noticed with the symptoms, there are actually a number of similarities between a cold and an allergy. The best way to determine if it is a common cold or allergies are how the symptoms occur. With allergies, the symptoms occur all at once. With a cold, the symptoms gradually occur, one at a time instead of all of them at one time.

Another way is the time of year. Winter is the most common time of year for colds while fall and spring can be the most common time for allergies. Finally, how long the allergies last will help you determine if you have allergies or a cold. Colds generally last a maximum of 10 days where allergies can last an entire season and usually only go away when you are away from the allergen.

How will my allergies be treated?

Most allergies are treated with avoidance; however, if you are unable to avoid the allergen, such as with dust, management techniques and medication are the only ways to treat the allergy.

If you haven't already, read the chapter on reducing allergens.

Can I outgrow my allergies?

While there are some studies that suggest long-term exposure to pet hair can reduce the number of allergic reactions you have, people do not outgrow their allergies. Once you have an allergy to dogs, you will always have an allergy to them; however, you may be able to build a resistance where you can live with a hypoallergenic breed.

Can you develop allergies?

Yes, allergies are something that can occur later in life, so while people may not have an allergy to dogs at a young age, they may develop it later in life.

Can moving to a different climate help my allergies?

While some people have experienced success with reducing their allergic reactions when they move to a different climate, it has not been successfully studied. In general, if you are still exposed to the allergen, you will still have the allergy.

For more information regarding allergies, please see the chapter on resources and contact an allergist near you.

2. FAQ about Dogs

Are dogs easy to train?

In general, yes, dogs are easy to train if you dedicate about 10 to 15 minutes of time each day. In addition, you will need to be consistent with training and with rules.

One thing that you should be aware of is that some dogs are more difficult to train than others, so make sure that you research the breed you are interested in.

Can you train an older dog?

The saying, "You can't teach an old dog new tricks," is actually a myth. Older dogs can be trained just as easily as a puppy, and all it takes is patience and consistency.

Adopting an older dog can be very rewarding, and while there will be some adjustment periods, the end result is a loving companion.

How old should a puppy be before it comes home?

This varies between breeders; however, the minimum age that you should take a puppy home is 8 weeks of age. The ideal age, however, is between 10 to 12 weeks of age. If your potential breeder wants you to take the puppy at 6 weeks or younger, find a different breeder. There are key developmental periods in that age group, and taking a puppy early can affect the puppy's development.

What sex is better? Male or female?

When it comes to the age old question of male or female, it really is up to your personal choice. Females tend to be more nurturing and patient with children; however, they also go through a lot of mood shifts.

Males are usually more dominant and will be more likely to wander away, but they are also more stable when it comes to emotions.

Most trainers will recommend a female for a first-time owner; however, I have found that every dog and person is different, so go with the sex that you feel comfortable with.

When can I start socializing my puppy?

Socialization actually starts the moment your puppy comes home as the puppy will socialize with you and your family. However, it is important to remember that you should wait for your dog to have its full series of vaccinations.

Should I neuter or spay my dog?

Yes, absolutely. There are many benefits to spaying and neutering, including protecting your dog from certain diseases. In addition, neutering and spaying often helps prevent certain behavior problems such as running away and dominance.

Is there a hypoallergenic breed that is better?

No. I would not recommend one hypoallergenic breed over another. Remember that a breed has to fit into your lifestyle so you should choose according to what you want.

In addition, the breeds listed in this book are the more popular hypoallergenic breeds and are in no way the better breeds. For some people, these breeds are, and for others, it may be a different breed all together.

Again, if you have any other questions about dogs, I recommend that you contact your potential breeder and discuss those questions with them.

Chapter Seven: Resources

While there are many resources out there for every single breed, I want to take the time to list a number of resources that will help you as a dog owner and also as someone who suffers from allergies.

1. Allergy Resources

There are many resources out there when you have allergies. You can start with any of these organizations; however, I strongly recommend that you start with your family doctor.

a) International Allergy Resources

ARIA: www.whiar.org

GINA: www.ginasthma.org

World Allergy Organization: www.worldallergy.org

INTERASMA: www.interasma.org

b) UK/Europe

Aha!: www.aha.ch

Allergy UK: www.allergyuk.org

Asthma Society of Ireland: www.asthma.ie

BSACI: www.bsaci.org

Danish Society for Allergology: danskallergi.dk

European Academy of Allergy and Clinical Immunology:
www.eaaci.org

European Federation for Allergy and Airway Diseases Patients
Association: www.efanet.org

Italian Federasma: www.federasmaeallergie.org

Finland Allergy and Asthma Association of Health:
www.allergia.fi

French Society of Allergology and Clinical Immunology:
www.lesallergies.fr

German Society for Allergology and Clinical Immunology:
dgaki.de

Nederlands Anafylaxis Netwerk: www.anafylaxis.nl

Norges Astma-og Allergiforbund: www.naaf.no

Polish Allergen Research Center: www.alergen.info.pl

Portuguese Society of Allergology: www.spaic.pt

Sociedad de Alergologos del Notre de Espana:
www.alergonorte.org

Societat Catalana d'Al-lergia i Immunologia Clinica:
www.scaic.cat

Sociedad Espanola de Alergologia e Immunologia Clinica:
www.seaic.es

Swedish Association for Allergology: www.sffa.nu

UCB Institute of Allergy: www.theucbinstituteofallergy.com

c) North America

AAN-MA: www.aanma.org

Allergist: http://www.acaai.org/allergist

Allergy Information Association: www.aaia.ca

American Academy of Allergy, Asthma and Immunology: www.aaaai.org

American College of Allergy, Asthma and Immunology: www.acaai.org

Anaphylaxis Network of Canada: www.anaphylaxis.org

AAFA: www.aafa.org

Asthma Society of Canada: www.asthma.ca

Asthma Kids Canada: www.asthmakids.ca

Canadian Society of Allergy and Clinical Immunology: csaci.ca

Clinical Immunology Society: www.clinimmsoc.org

FOCiS: www.focisnet.org

NIAID: www.niaid.nih.gov

2. Recommended Books on Allergies

Although this book offers you a lot of information regarding battling your allergies, I recommend that you read some of the books before you bring home a hypoallergenic puppy. This will give you a better understanding of what allergies are and also how to combat them.

Allergies A to Z By Myron A. Lipkowitz, RP, MD
Facts On File, Inc.

Allergy, Asthma and Immunology From Infancy to Adulthood By Warren Bieman, et al.

Best Guide to Allergy By Nathan Schultz, Allan Giannini, Terrace Chang

Complete Book of Children's Allergies By B.R. Feldman, MD

Sinus Survival: A Self-Help Guide for Allergies, Bronchitis, Colds and Sinusitis
By Robert S. Ivker

Sneezing Your Head Off? How to Live With Your Allergic Nose
By Peter Boggs, MD

Taming Asthma and Allergy By Controlling Your Environment
By Robert A. Wood, MD

You Can Do Something About Your Allergies
By Nelson L. Novick

3. Resources for Dog Owners

Not only should you have resources for your allergies, but you should have a number of resources for your dog. I recommend joining an online group for your dog breed, there are thousands of them out there, to connect with other like-minded people.

In addition to the dog groups, keep these resources handy.

a) Kennel Clubs

American Kennel Club: www.akc.org

Australian National Kennel Council: www.ankc.org.au

Canadian Kennel Club: www.ckc.ca

Danish Kennel Club: www.dkk.dk

English Kennel Club: www.thekennelclub.org.uk

Estonian Kennel Union: kennelliit.ee

FCI: www.fci.be

Finnish Kennel Club: www.kennelliitto.fi

French Kennel Club: www.scc.asso.fr

German Kennel Club: www.vdh.de

Italian Kennel Club: www.enci.it

Irish Kennel Club: www.ikc.ie

Japan Kennel Club: www.jkc.or.jp

New Zealand Kennel Club: www.nzkc.org.nz

Norwegian Kennel Club: www.nkk.no

Swedish Kennel Club: www.skk.se

Swiss Kennel Club: www.skg.ch

b) Dog Owner Resources

Best Friends: bestfriends.org

Breeder.net: www.breeders.net

Dogs Trust: www.dogstrust.org.uk

Pet360: www.pet360.com

RSPCA: www.rspca.org.uk

Vetmedicine: vetmedicine.about.com

4. Personal Notes

This section is designed for you to make your own notes in regards to questions to ask the breeder and to help answer the many questions throughout the choosing the right breed chapter.

_____

_____

_____

_____

_____

_____

_____

_____

_____

_____

_____

_____

_____

_____

_____

_____

_____

_____

_____

_____

_____

_____

_____

_____

_____

_____

_____

_____
_____
_____
_____
_____
_____
_____
_____
_____
_____
_____
_____
_____
_____
_____
_____
_____
_____
_____
_____
_____
_____
_____
_____
_____
_____
_____
_____
_____
_____
_____
_____
_____

9 780993 004322